Arts-Based Approaches to Promote Mental Health and Well-Being

This book provides insights on how creative and expressive approaches can promote psychosocial well-being among children, youth, and their caregivers living in conditions of adversity around the world.

Arts-based psychosocial approaches give children a means to tap into their strengths as well as adaptively communicate and process experiences in ways that promote their own and overall family well-being. Offering an overview of the impact of adverse childhood experiences on lifelong health and functioning and how arts-based approaches can be protective, this book discusses relevant theory and research, as well as case studies and findings from mixed methods program evaluations. Examples from the Healing and Education Through the Arts (HEART) initiative from Save the Children are discussed in depth, and demonstrate the benefits of creative self-expression among children and families in the most challenging environments around the world.

Creative arts therapists, public health professionals, education specialists, policymakers, and humanitarian groups seeking to provide cost-effective support to communities in need will find, in this book, insights on the impact of large-scale arts-based interventions in a range of public health and education settings.

Sara Hommel leads the global Mental Health and Psychosocial Support portfolio, including the Healing and Education through the Arts program, for Save the Children's International Department of Education and Child Protection.

Girija Kaimal is Professor and Chair of the Creative Arts Therapies department at Drexel University. Her research examines the physiological and psychological health outcomes of creative visual and narrative self-expression.

Arts-Based Approaches to Promote Mental Health and Well-Being

Supporting Children and Families in Conditions of Adversity

Edited by
Sara Hommel and Girija Kaimal

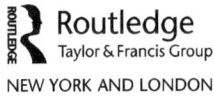
Routledge
Taylor & Francis Group

NEW YORK AND LONDON

Designed cover image: Photo by Sara Hommel

First published 2025
by Routledge
605 Third Avenue, New York, NY 10158

and by Routledge
4 Park Square, Milton Park, Abingdon, Oxon, OX14 4RN

Routledge is an imprint of the Taylor & Francis Group, an informa business

ISBN: 9781032434810 (hbk)
ISBN: 9781032434803 (pbk)
ISBN: 9781003367529 (ebk)

DOI: 10.4324/9781003367529

Typeset in Times New Roman
by Newgen Publishing UK

Contents

Acknowledgments

The editors would like to thank the many people who played a vital role in the development of the HEART program. There are too many to list, but in addition to those who are co-authors of this book, we would also like to extend special thanks to Maria Regina Alfonso and Audrey Di Maria. We also thank the thousands of HEART facilitators around the world who bring arts-based psychosocial support to children and families every day.

We would also like to thank Charlene Engelhard and the Charles Engelhard Foundation for their championship of HEART.

The co-authors of the book would like to thank the many colleagues who contributed to the case examples, monitoring and evaluation reports, and other sources that contributed to this volume. This includes Edlira Ngjeci and the Save the Children Albania team, Valid Zhubi and the Save the Children Kosovo team, Brilanda Ballata and the Handikos team, Betty Namugga and Kevin Mubuke and the Save the Children Uganda team, Bram Marantika and the Save the Children Indonesia team, Reem Ibrahim and Reem Joudieh and the Save the Children Lebanon team, Widad Ezzo, Yussef Muhammed, Samia Ali and the Save the Children Syria team, Adenike Webb, and Pamela Fried.

In addition, we would like to thank Kristyn S. Stickley for her creative illustrations, and Iain Hinchliffe for his support with photos and figures.

Author Biographies

Carolyn Alesbury is a Basic Education Senior Advisor at Save the Children. Since joining the organization in 2010, Carolyn has supported education programs across a range of contexts and regions, including both humanitarian and development settings. Her primary area of focus is inclusive education for children with disabilities, and she is a co-founder and co-lead of the organization's global Inclusive Education Community of Practice. She also serves as a global HEART trainer and supported the adaptation and launch of HEART for All Children in 2016. Carolyn previously worked as a middle school special education paraprofessional in the United States, and holds a Doctorate in Education Policy from The George Washington University, as well as Masters degrees in both Human Rights and Education. Her doctoral research focused on the role of schools in strengthening social cohesion.

May Aoun is a global Senior Mental Health and Psychosocial Support (MHPSS) Advisor at Save the Children. She has extensive experience supporting comprehensive MHPSS strategies and interventions, and designing, facilitating, and evaluating MHPSS programs, in several countries and regions. Prior to joining Save the Children, May supported MHPSS programs and research at War Child Holland. May has co-led several national, regional, and global MHPSS working groups and inter-agency task forces. She is interested in the intricate connections between mental health and creative expression. She firmly believes that art can communicate emotions, inspire self-reflection, and promote healing in ways that classical therapeutic approaches often cannot. During her time at Save the Children, she has supported the design, adaptation, and implementation of several arts-based MHPSS programs. May holds a Master of Arts in Clinical Psychology from the Lebanese University.

Asli Arslanbek is an artist, art therapist, and Assistant Professor of Art Therapy at The University of Tampa. She holds a PhD in Creative Arts Therapies from Drexel University and a Master of Arts in Art Therapy from New York

University. Her primary interest lies in utilizing arts-based approaches to enhance mental health and well-being among diverse populations, including a particular interest in international art therapy and community-based art therapy practices. As part of her doctoral research, she explored the characteristics of art therapists' efforts to build capacity in humanitarian emergency settings. Aside from her professional pursuits, Asli currently resides in Tampa, Florida with her husband, toddler daughter and her beloved dog, Maya.

Aida Bekic is a global Senior MHPSS Advisor at Save the Children. She has more than 20 years of experience in regional Child Protection and global Mental Health and Psychosocial Support programming. In her current role, she supports MHPSS for children and families in multiple countries in Eastern Europe, the Middle East, Africa, and Asia. Aida has a particular interest in the protection and well-being of children with disabilities and has supported multiple disability support initiatives across Eastern Europe. Aida holds a Master of Arts in Sociology from the University of Sarajevo. Her Master's thesis focused on the Social Causes of Trafficking for Women and Children and her related work supporting the protection of children and families has supported national anti-trafficking strategies in Bosnia and Herzegovina, and other countries in Eastern Europe.

Rebekka Dieterich-Hartwell is a dance/movement therapist in Philadelphia. She has over 20 years of clinical experience with adults with acute and chronic mental illnesses, substance abuse issues, eating disorders, and psychological trauma. Her research interests are threefold: in the area of psychological trauma with a specific focus on the neurobiological effects of PTSD, in the connection between music and movement and the selection process of music for dance/movement therapy sessions with different populations, and in using dance and movement as an acculturation resource for refugees, asylees, and immigrants. She holds a PhD in Creative Arts Therapies from Drexel University. Rebekka is currently a postdoctoral research fellow in the creative arts therapy department at Drexel University and serves as Member at Large (Eastern Region) on the Board of the American Dance Therapy Association.

Sara Hommel has more than 25 years of experience in global development and humanitarian response. She currently leads the global MHPSS portfolio for Save the Children's International Department of Education and Child Protection. Prior to joining Save the Children, Sara spent several years at the Brookings Institution where she designed and managed research and advocacy on global education policy and practice. Before her time at Brookings, she worked with several non-governmental organizations addressing the needs of children affected by conflict and poverty in multiple countries. Sara holds degrees in Sociology and International Relations from St. Lawrence University and Central European University and is a doctoral candidate at the UCL Institute of Education (IOE) at the University of London. Her research focuses on the impact of school based psychosocial support programming for children affected by multiple adversities.

Girija Kaimal is Professor and Chair of the Creative Arts Therapies department at the Drexel University College of Nursing and Health Professions. In her Health, Arts, Learning and Evaluation (HALE) research lab, she examines the physiological and psychological health outcomes of visual and narrative self-expression. She has published extensively, including a book with Oxford University Press called *The Expressive Instinct*. Her current research examines outcomes of art therapy for military service members with traumatic brain injury and post-traumatic stress, and arts-based approaches to mitigate chronic stress among patients and caregivers in pediatric hematology/oncology units. Additional international research projects include examining the therapeutic underpinnings of indigenous and traditional artforms and creative self-expression in times of adversity across the human lifespan. Girija holds a doctorate from the Harvard University Graduate School of Education, Master of Arts from Drexel University, and Bachelor's in Design from the National Institute of Design in India.

Ana Lagidze has more than two decades of experience in supporting national and regional education initiatives with non-governmental organizations, public sector institutions, UNICEF, and Save the Children. Ana has supported inclusive education strategies, teacher training initiatives, and education certification mechanisms for both the early education and primary education sectors in multiple countries. Ana holds a Master of Arts in Education from Harvard University. In her current role, Ana serves as the Early Childhood Care and Development (ECCD) Expert for Save the Children in Georgia where she oversees the development of education program strategies and partnerships for multiple national education initiatives. Ana has a special interest in inclusive education and multi-sector disability support programming and oversaw one of the first pilots of HEART for All Children in Georgia.

Dario Lipovac is a global Senior Advisor for Mental Health and Psychosocial Support at Save the Children where he has worked to support local, regional, and global MHPSS strategies and approaches for more than a decade. In his current role, he supports HEART and related MHPSS programming for children and families in more than ten countries in Europe, Africa, Asia, and the Middle East. Dario holds a Master of Arts in Psychology from the University of Banja Luka and a Cognitive Behavioral Therapy (CBT) Certification from the European Association for Behavioural and Cognitive Therapies. Dario is passionate about promoting evidence-based, accessible, and transformative approaches to support the mental health and psychosocial well-being of children and adults around the world, through expressive arts-based approaches and CBT.

Bani Malhotra is a Board-Certified, Registered Art Therapist and Postdoctoral Fellow at Virginia Commonwealth University. She serves as an interventionist and researcher for the Resources for Enhancing All Caregivers' Health – REACH TBI project, an evidence-based telehealth intervention study for caregivers of Traumatic Brain Injury. Her research focuses on interdisciplinary approaches to developing and implementing psychosocial recovery and rehabilitation interventions in the context of adversity, stress, injury, and illness. She holds a PhD in Creative Arts Therapies from Drexel University, a Master's Degree in Art Therapy from The George Washington University, and a Master's Degree in Psychology from the University of Delhi. She has extensive experience working with individuals across the lifespan in medical, forensic, psychiatric, and school settings in India and the United States. She currently chairs the American Art Therapy Association's International Shared Interest Group.

Phoebe Marabi has over 15 years of experience in humanitarian and global development child protection programming. She is currently a Senior Advisor for Child Protection at Save the Children where she has led multiple child protection approaches in humanitarian responses across disaster and conflict settings in the Middle East, West Africa, East and Southern Africa, and Latin America, and supported global development work with initiatives addressing the needs of homeless children, Orphans and Vulnerable Children, Child Labour, and Counter Trafficking strategies. She holds a Diploma in Social Work from the Institute of Community Development in Nairobi, Kenya, a Higher Diploma in Psychological Counselling from the Kenya Institute of Professional Counselling, and a Master's Degree in Advanced Child Protection from the University of Kent in the United Kingdom.

Miroslava Marjanovic is an integrative psychotherapist for children and youth in Bosnia and Herzegovina. She holds a Master of Arts in Social Psychology from the University of Belgrade and a Psychotherapy Certification from the Association for Integrative Child and Adolescent Psychotherapy in Bosnia and Herzegovina. Miroslava has extensive experience working with children and youth affected by adversity, including as a kindergarten and elementary school counselor, in a local NGO focused on improving access to education for children from vulnerable groups, with Save the Children as a Mental Health and Psychosocial Support Specialist, and in private counseling and psychotherapy practice focused on supporting children and families with special needs. She is interested in art-based therapy that integrates reflective self-awareness with creative emotional expression to support children's mental health.

Jean Nkhonjera is a Technical Advisor for ECCD at Save the Children in Malawi. She holds a Bachelor of Arts in Education from the University of Malawi and is currently studying for a Master of Arts in Education Policy, Planning, and Leadership. In her current role at Save the Children, Jean supports early education programming, education policy development, community partnerships, and parent support initiatives in Malawi. Jean has supported the integration of MHPSS, including HEART, into the early and primary education systems in Malawi, serving as a HEART trainer and program technical focal point. Jean has a particular interest in School Readiness, Social Emotional Learning, Disability Inclusion, and ECCD in emergencies.

Amy Parker is a Senior Learning through Play Advisor for Save the Children. In her current role, she supports education teams to deepen play-based approaches to improve holistic outcomes for children in different contexts around the world. Amy initially trained as a secondary school teacher in the UK and worked in schools in Bradford and London. She holds a Bachelor of Arts in Modern Foreign Languages from Durham University and a Post Graduate Certificate in Education from the University of Leeds. She has worked in international development for more than 15 years, including with multiple international non-governmental organizations, with a major focus on fragile and conflict affected settings. Amy is also active in several international education networks, including the Inter-Agency Network for Education in Emergencies and the UK Education and Development Forum, holding leadership roles such as working group and conference co-chair.

Laila Sabbagh is a Mental Health and Psychosocial Support Senior Leader at Save the Children in Mexico. Her work focuses on the integration of Mental Health and Psychosocial Support in education and social support programs in Mexico. In her current role, she oversees the integration of HEART and complementary MHPSS programs into preschools, primary schools, and community centers across several regions in Mexico and also supports MHPSS integration in several other countries in Central and South America. Laila holds a Master of Arts in Psychology from the Metropolitan Autonomous University and a Master of Arts in Applied Linguistics from the National Autonomous University of Mexico.

Victoria Schwachter is currently a Project Coordinator at Drexel University where she supports the operations of the Creative Arts Therapies Department guided by her 20 years of work as an art therapist. Victoria's public service work, which began in special education in 1990, has spanned elementary through high school settings and has included psychiatric residences, inpatient units, and partial hospitalization settings. Concentrations in trauma sensitive care, perspective-taking, self-expression, and cognitive flexibility have helped her hold nonjudgmental space for people living with anxiety, PTSD, autism, mood disorders and accompanying high-risk situations such as self-injury and suicidal thoughts and behaviors. She holds a Master of Arts in Art Therapy from Drexel University. Victoria's current interests include deconstructing Eurocentric definitions of health and healing, and her enduring wish for the natural inclusion of the expressive arts in our collective response to life.

Kristyn S. Stickley is a Board-Certified, Registered Art Therapist and a Licensed Professional Clinical Counselor in the state of Minnesota. Kristyn received her Master's Degree from Drexel University in Art Therapy & Counseling in 2019. She has worked in medical, inpatient psychiatric, community mental health, residential, school, and outpatient settings. Kristyn is currently enrolled in Drexel University's PhD in Creative Arts Therapies program, where she works as a Research Fellow in the HALE Lab. She also has a professional background in illustration and works as a Graphic Recorder using words and symbols to capture visual representations of group processes, assisting groups in identifying new insights and alternate ways of understanding their situations.

Introduction

Purpose of Writing this Book

Our main purpose in writing this book was to share lessons learned from the successful implementation of the Healing and Education through the Arts (HEART) program worldwide. We sought to document and share how creative self-expression can be a foundation for mental health and well-being.

Arts-based psychosocial support offers an opportunity to enhance well-being and fill critical gaps in mental health and psychosocial support services for children, families, and communities around the world. The arts can be a creative, fun, and interactive mechanism to support children's psychosocial well-being, learning, and development and are a particularly effective approach to supporting children affected by adversity. By integrating into existing child support settings, with existing child support workers, arts-based psychosocial support can be a cost-effective approach to improving psychosocial well-being across the globe.

In this book, we seek to share experiences of one of the largest arts-based public health programs supporting children, families, and communities in global development and humanitarian response programming worldwide, HEART, at the international non-governmental organization Save the Children. Over the last decade, the HEART program has supported more than one million children, as well as parents, caregivers, and staff, across 30 countries.

HEART is a demonstrated example of a scalable and adaptable approach to arts-based psychosocial support. The HEART program was developed from the knowledge and experience of the clinical professions of creative and expressive arts therapies and has since been adapted to offer non-clinical mental health support strategies to teachers, facilitators, and caregivers to manage stress, improve self-regulation, communicate, play, and learn from the arts.

This book is an edited volume on effective and scalable arts-based approaches to promote psychosocial well-being among children, youth, and their caregivers living in conditions of adversity around the world. It offers an overview of the impact of adverse childhood experiences on lifelong health and functioning and how arts-based approaches can be protective, preventative, and curative.

DOI: 10.4324/9781003367529-1

Arts-based psychosocial approaches offer children a means to tap into their strengths as well as adaptively communicate and process experiences in ways that promote their well-being.

One of the challenges of arts-based therapeutic intervention work is scalability and lack of trained clinicians. The plan to write this book began over a series of conversations between the editors on sharing lessons learned from the challenges and successes of implementing and scaling the HEART program. By bringing together educators, researchers, and practitioners, we sought to share both the science of arts-based interventions as well as insights gained from implementation across a range of sites around the world. In particular, given the thoughtful adaptations made with HEART across the world and with different constituents, we wanted to share lessons learned on how to address the public health needs of psychosocial support, including for children, of all ages and abilities, their families and communities.

In this book we offer the science as well as case examples and mixed methods program evaluations to show how to effectively conduct a model of practice that helps bring sustainable programming benefits of creative self-expression among children and youth in the most challenging environments around the world. We expect that this book will be of interest to public health professionals, health providers, mental health and social work communities, educators, policy makers, and global development and humanitarian groups seeking to provide cost-effective psychosocial supports to communities in need. Our aim is to share how the therapeutic underpinnings of expressive and creative arts therapies can be developed and adapted successfully into non-clinical public health, education, and humanitarian realms.

This book is co-authored by 17 professionals including academics and practitioners involved in the design, delivery, and research of arts-based psychosocial support interventions. The co-authors bring diverse experience of working in art-based psychosocial support in multiple countries and programming contexts, and collectively originate from 11 countries including Bosnia and Herzegovina, Georgia, Germany, India, Kenya, Lebanon, Malawi, Mexico, Turkey, the United Kingdom, and the United States. The contributors to this volume participated pro bono and committed to their chapters from a deep sense belief and lived experiences of the impact of arts-based programming to help support children, families, and communities affected by adversity. The co-authors commitment to writing this book comes from the desire to share these effective lessons learned with a wider audience.

Values, Worldview, and Approach to Arts-based Psychosocial Support

Why arts-based approaches: As humans we are wired to be empathic and inherently led to care for those in need. Humanitarian organizations work to support communities facing adversities most often in the form of financial aid and material resources. The approach of giving aid is often led by ensuring that physical and physiological needs are met. In addition, organizations might offer programming for psychological support in the form of interventions and programming largely defined by Western paradigms of therapy. What if instead of these external drops, the approach to responding to adversities delved into our creative and expressive instincts deeply rooted in our human evolutionary history.

Creativity is a defining feature of the human species. Living with the reality of uncertainty in our human lives, our inherent creative capacity, which can manifest itself in many ways in our lives, is the source of our ability to survive and thrive. The desire to express ourselves is an innate need, that serves as a safety valve for health and well-being. As humans we seek to share what we know in order to maximize our survival and enable a sense of belonging of our unique selves in an accepting community of peers. We have evolved arts practices over time and the future promises to bring new tools for research and self-expression.

Beyond literal self-expression, creative self-expression is especially relevant because it gives us an outlet, a perspective, and thus a sense of agency and control. Most scholarship about art has tended to be about viewing art or experiencing it, especially the works of famous artists. We cannot live out every life scenario and therefore receptive artistic expressive experiences such as encountering the stories embedded in artistic works of paintings, fiction, poetry, drama, and dance help us learn vicariously about life and all that can be. Expressive artistic works enable us to add the stories of our own experiences into this pantheon of creative works. By tapping into the arts, we tap into a global resource that has evolved and exists everywhere in the world.

Role of families, caregivers and communities in caring for children: Children by virtue of their developmental stage are associated with the adults and caregivers around them. These might be older children and youth, parents, and other care providers. Adversities affect not just children, but the adults in their families, schools, and communities. To support and care for the psychosocial needs of adults in a community is essential for the well-being of the children in their care. The ways in which parents, caregivers, and staff in humanitarian organizations can be supported such that they can better manage adversities for their own well-being while also supporting growing children, is an important dimension of sustainable care.

Range of arts practices. In this book, we refer to the expressive arts broadly and include references to visual arts, music, dance, poetry and prose, movement, and drama. The arts are present worldwide in every human community and the way they manifests varies. Thus, we refer to artistic practices broadly and distinguish unique attributes of each as they pertain to research findings and context of practice. There are a range of arts integrated professions, including arts health practitioners, arts facilitators, teaching artists, and expressive arts therapists. The work done in HEART is led by facilitators trained to support the psychosocial needs of children and adults in non-clinical health settings such as schools or community centers, and thus are often teachers, school counselors, and community center facilitators.

Context of arts-based psychosocial support: We acknowledge that the HEART initiative developed from a clinical foundation in expressive and creative arts therapies. This means that the idea that the arts can be therapeutic emerges in the Western world from the disciplines of art therapy, music therapy, dance movement therapy, drama therapy, and poetry therapy. These disciplines together constitute the creative arts therapies. Although the arts have been part of human existence for as long as homo sapiens have lived, the professionalization of the use of the arts for mental health and well-being is a development of the mid-twentieth century.

In addition to the influence of the creative arts therapies, HEART integrates principles of social work and public health that recognize the role of communities of care and support in children's development. The social and ecological context of a child's development in their communities (home, school, society) are considered with care and sensitivity in HEART programming. We recognize these distinctions and highlight how the work of HEART is adapted to different global contexts of adversity and are responsive to local context, resources, and needs. HEART is explicitly not therapy or clinical mental health services, rather efforts to promote health and well-being informed by the clinical foundations of creative and expressive arts therapies.

Research and evaluation with children and youth: Throughout the book, we share current research on the role of the arts in enhancing well-being for children, caregivers, and communities. Research in the HEART program has mainly occurred in the form of program evaluations of efforts around the world. These include qualitative, quasi-experimental, and mixed methods social science study designs. The evaluations have used innovative local data collection tools, and also ensured that data collectors and analysts were recruited locally and actively involved in all aspects of the evaluations. Culture and context-specific considerations for research and evaluation are a priority for HEART. Many standardized measures are not necessarily applicable in all local contexts and as such, HEART programs have found qualitative approaches of interviews and focus groups to be more meaningful and culturally relevant as a form of gathering data and understanding the impacts of the programs.

Rights-based foundation: As an initiative of Save the Children, the HEART program is grounded in the UN Convention on the Rights of the Child. All children have the right to freedom of expression (Article 13), education in a spirit of peace and tolerance (Articles 28–29), play (Article 31), and psychological recovery and reintegration if they are victims of abuse or armed conflicts (Article 39). These rights apply to all children, regardless of gender, ethnic or linguistic background, disability status, religion, or other factors, including refugee status. Additional treaties also recognize the rights of specific groups of people, including individuals at risk of racial discrimination, women and girls, migrant workers, and persons with disabilities. Save the Children prioritizes working with children who are most at risk of their rights not being fulfilled and is continuously reviewing and improving the package to better meet the needs of specific populations.

Limitations: In writing this book, we also want to acknowledge the essential boundaries and limitations of the work. The group of authors who contributed to this book range from creative art therapists, arts researchers, psychologists, sociologists, social workers, education professionals, and humanitarian workers. This diversity in experience is beneficial as HEART is a multi-disciplinary approach and we also acknowledge that the perspectives we share are necessarily defined by our own professional experiences and as such are constrained by what we know and have learned over time. We do not claim to represent everything that is known or all aspects of arts-based psychosocial support for children and communities living in adversity. We have, however, tried to present the current state of the literature and our reflections of practices and approaches to research that represent current knowledge and awareness.

Overview of Chapters

Our first chapter provides an overview of the history of the HEART program at Save the Children, from the first stages of program design and piloting to review, revision, and standardization of a global approach, to where the program is today. The second and third chapters review the theory and research that informed the design of HEART, with special attention to the impact of adversity on child development and well-being, and the role of the arts in supporting children and adults affected by adversity. The fourth chapter reviews the HEART program in detail, including the influence of the creative arts therapies on the design of the program and the ethical standards within in, the content of HEART sessions, the logistics of launching the program in a new location, the process of training facilitators and delivering the program to children and adults, adaptations of the program to different contexts and populations, the program's approach to monitoring and evaluation, and varied types of program utilization in the global development and humanitarian response sectors.

The second part of the book (Chapters 5–10) offers more focused exploration of different aspects of the HEART program. Chapter 5 explores the use of the program with an early childhood age group (preschool age range) and Chapter 6 explores HEART programming for children in primary and secondary school age groups. Chapter 7 looks at the adaptation of HEART to support children with disabilities while Chapter 8 looks at the use of the program to support parents and caregivers, Chapter 9 explores the experience of using HEART to support staff well-being, and Chapter 10 offers insights into the experience of scaling the program with local partners. Chapters 5–10 all offer overviews of their key topics alongside practical case examples of the program's experience in different contexts and locations around the world. Chapter 11 reflects on lessons learned from challenges and successes over the last decade of global HEART experience, highlights the importance of HEART champions (advocates), and offers expectations about the future of HEART.

Key Takeaways

This chapter provided an overview of our motivations to write this book, including from personal experiences as practitioners, clinicians, and researchers. We introduce the ideas of the value of the arts in promoting psychosocial well-being worldwide for children and adults in communities affected by adversity. The structure of the book and how we link the science and practice of art-based psychosocial support are included.

Chapter 1

Healing and Education Through the Arts at Save the Children

Sara Hommel, May Aoun, Aida Bekic, and Dario Lipovac

Save the Children is an international nongovernmental organization that supports children's health, education, and protection in 115 countries around the world. One key aspect of this work includes a focus on the psychosocial well-being of children, the goal being to ensure that children's psychological and social needs are addressed as part of a comprehensive approach to supporting children's development and well-being globally.

In 2008, after decades of ad hoc approaches to addressing children's psychosocial well-being, Save the Children decided to develop a standardized approach to psychosocial support. Over the course of several years, the organization undertook consultations with child development experts from multiple countries and multiple sectors, including those from the fields of social work, psychology, education, and public health. Within these consultations, the role of the arts kept surfacing as an important approach for supporting child development and psychosocial well-being. Art therapists and other expressive arts practitioners proposed numerous methods and approaches for integrating expressive arts into Save the Children's work. To figure out what could work and how best it could be operationalized within the organization's existing programming, a series of approaches were tested in different countries. These pilot programs included a range of activities from focused art therapy approaches (including the support of consultant art therapists) to recreational arts-based activities intended to engage children in fun and creativity in safe environments away from violence and other stressors in the local community. After one year of piloting multiple approaches, Save the Children consulted with the stakeholders involved, including the child support staff who organized and facilitated the activities and the children who participated. The results led the organization to conclude that expressive arts are a good approach for integrating psychosocial support into its global work and that the most appropriate way to do it would be a focused, nonspecialized model that does not require art therapists or other mental health professionals but rather utilizes the methods and techniques of the creative arts therapies to inform existing child support settings such as classrooms or community-based spaces where non-mental-health professionals support children on a regular basis.

DOI: 10.4324/9781003367529-2

After reviewing the pilot programs, Save the Children confirmed its intention to develop a standardized approach to arts-based psychosocial support and focused on organizing global experts to collaboratively develop a standardized and adaptable program model while also fund-raising to test this new approach in different settings around the world. It is important to note that the process of developing the program was a global initiative from the start. Over the course of several years, from 2011 to 2015, a group of global experts including art therapists, education specialists, social workers, psychologists, and public health specialists from eight different countries[1] consulted, designed, reviewed, redesigned, and tested multiple approaches to integrating structured expressive arts activities into classrooms and community-based child support spaces. They designed different types of activities informed by the methods and techniques of the creative arts therapies and designed different approaches to training non-mental-health specialists to facilitate these activities with children of different ages in different contexts. The model developed as one in which those delivering the program to children are mostly non-mental-health professionals such as teachers or community facilitators who receive ongoing support from local supervisors who are Mental Health and Psychosocial Support (MHPSS) professionals.

Once the standardized model was in place in 2016, it ran for two years and then underwent a global review that collected feedback (documented best practices and recommendations for adjustments) from program trainers, facilitators, and supervisors. The global review led to a program update (revised program support materials, updated training protocol, and adjusted monitoring and evaluation guidance) that was standardized and launched in 2018. The result of this process is Save the Children's Healing and Education through the Arts (HEART) global arts-based psychosocial support program.

HEART was initially designed to support children between the ages of 4 to 18. It eventually expanded to support their parents and caregivers as well as their teachers and community-based facilitators (and other child support workers such as social workers and health workers). Supporting children in contexts of adversity should include both direct support to children and support for the adults in their lives because the adversity experienced by children affects the entire community. Strategies for improving the well-being of children should focus on the entire community and all the spaces and people responsible for supporting children's development, learning, and well-being. Specifics about the experience of the program model for different age groups and different contexts are explored in more detail in Chapters 4–10.

The Local Context

In most of the settings where Save the Children works, mental health services are limited. Most schools do not have professional counselors such as trained social workers or psychologists, and mental health services outside the school or community-based child support spaces are limited (either due to few existing local service providers or limited access for those unable to pay for private services). Providing nonspecialized MHPSS through schools or community-based centers, delivered by non-mental-health providers such as teachers or community facilitators, is one way to support children affected by stress in their current context as well as a method for interrupting the potential long-term impact that such stress might have on their future mental and physical health. The mitigating psychosocial support provided through HEART and comparable nonclinical approaches to MHPSS can have both immediate and long-term benefits.

The HEART program is intended to support all children in the classroom or community-based center. Children are not selected to participate but rather the entire class or center-based group is organized to participate regularly in HEART activities. As a focused nonspecialized MHPSS approach, HEART relies on a broader framework of MHPSS services and supports, including local referral mechanisms that link individual children in need of specialized clinical mental health support with appropriate services that exist outside programs supported by Save the Children (often provided through the local health-care system or by international clinical health nongovernmental organizations operating in the local context when the local system is stretched by an emergency such as a natural disaster or armed conflict).

The locations prioritized for HEART programming are those in which children are affected by multiple stressors and adverse conditions such as poverty, natural disasters, armed conflict, disease, and displacement. The HEART program recognizes that children can be affected by community-level stressors (such as an adverse event that impacts an entire community) as well as by personal stressors (such as those related to personal or family-level experiences). The activities within the program are intended to support children to explore and process feelings, emotions, and ideas related to multiple aspects of their lives, including both personal and community-level experiences.

The local programming contexts in which HEART is used can be categorized as both "humanitarian" (or emergency response) as well as "development." Within global development and humanitarian response programming, these terms are used to delineate between programming that supports a specific crisis ("humanitarian" or "emergency") such as an armed conflict or natural disaster and programming that supports settings affected by chronic adversities ("development") such as extreme poverty. Save the Children uses HEART in both humanitarian and development settings. It also uses the program in contexts referred to as **nexus settings**, meaning locations in which there is ongoing or recurrent transition between humanitarian and development programming. Because many of Save the Children's local programming contexts regularly shift between these categorizations, this terminology is mostly administrative, often used to categorize the logistical aspects of programming and the funding sources dedicated to it.

One of the most important aspects of the HEART program is its adaptability to different contexts and conditions. HEART is designed to be a standardized structured program, but many aspects of that design allow it to be customized to the local setting to address local needs and incorporate local cultural arts traditions to strengthen the artistic experience and the connection of the program to the local setting. This approach can mean adapting specific activities to address specific situations, scheduling sessions to adapt to local events, and using local arts traditions for fun and engaging activities. The local arts traditions that are added in the local context most often relate to the use of music and dance that is often already known to the children, thus adding a fun and familiar local activity that serves to both energize and ground participation in the structured program. This local adaptability allows the program to integrate into the classroom or community-based center in a way that is gentle and sustainable, building on existing activities and traditions, becoming part of the school or center environment.

In most settings, HEART is integrated into the classroom or center through weekly sessions that take place over several months. On average, HEART sessions are designed for a 1-hour or 1.5-hour period. The duration of the program varies from one location to another based on the existing local programming structure. For example, when HEART is integrated into a school, HEART sessions are scheduled to take place once or twice per week in each classroom for the entire school year. In a location with a nine-month school year, the duration of one HEART program cycle would be approximately nine months. When HEART is integrated into a local community-based center in which children attend activities for six months of the year, the duration of the HEART program cycle would be approximately six months. When integrated into a school, the intention is for the program to recur year after year, meaning many children attend the program for more than one year as they would participate at different grade levels in the school. When integrated into a community-based center, the intention is for the program to recur for as long as the center is functional and focused on providing programming for children. So, if a community-based center is established to respond to a specific situation (such as a natural disaster or armed conflict), HEART would be intended to continue for as long as the center is operational, which could be several months or several years, so the HEART program cycle could be as short as four months or as long as 12 months (per cohort), depending on how the programming is organized in that space.

The number of children who participate in a HEART session at one time is determined by the local setting. If there are 30 children in a classroom, all 30 children should participate in HEART regularly. Some sessions would be facilitated to include all 30 children at once, and some sessions would be organized in smaller groups such as two groups of 15 each. Depending on how many trained HEART facilitators are available (often teachers) and the available physical space, these two smaller groups could participate in parallel sessions or could be scheduled for different session times within the week. Often in classroom settings, the split group option results in one group doing HEART in their classroom while the other group goes outside or to another location in the school for an alternate activity (e.g., game, sport). This pattern is repeated later in the week to ensure that both groups participate in the HEART session.[2]

The most important aspect of the logistics of the groups is that the groups are consistent for the duration of the program cycle, meaning that the same children participate in the same group over time. This approach ensures a process of group bonding, empathy building, and group support (children become supportive of themselves and of each other). For classrooms, this grouping is a natural process because the children in the classroom are usually a consistent group for the entire school year. For community-based centers, this grouping can require some logistical coordination to schedule groups of the same children to meet weekly over time if the existing programming is not already organized for consistent grouping (often organized by age group).

The HEART Program

HEART is designed to provide weekly sessions over extended periods (such as nine months when following the school year). Two specific types of sessions are organized: structured sessions and open sessions. If HEART sessions are organized twice per week in the local setting, one session is a structured session, and one is an open session. If HEART sessions are organized once per week, then the structured and open sessions alternate.[3] The **structured sessions** are predesigned to focus on a specific topic or theme and use a specific art form to represent personal or group reflections on that topic or theme. The **open sessions** are predesigned to use a specific art form without any facilitator guidance so that the art-making part of the session is open for the participants to create art, using the specific art form of that session, in any way they like without any guidance, around a specific topic or theme. In both types of sessions, the session starts with an arts-based relaxation activity and finishes with an arts-based grounding activity. Between the two is the art-making and sharing circle, through which children create art and are then invited to share it, visually or verbally (or both), with their peers and facilitators. It is this combination of activities across a session that produces the holistic impact that HEART aims to achieve.

Components of a Standard HEART Session

A standard HEART session lasts 1 to 1.5 hours and comprises the following components: relaxation activity; introduction to thematic topic (structured session) or introduction to open art making; art making; sharing circle; and a grounding activity.

Relaxation activities include short-term activities intended to promote physical and mental relaxation. These mostly involve dramatic play, music, dance, or other body movement approaches that promote muscle relaxation and controlled breathing. Examples include dramatic play activities that facilitate either muscle tensing and relaxing, such as pretending to pick fruit off a tree, squeezing the fruit in the hands (muscle tensing), and then tossing the fruit on the ground (muscle relaxing), or controlled breathing such as pretending to smell something nice and then gently blowing something away. Over time, these activities become tools to support stress processing and emotional regulation.

Art-making activities include the use of drawing, painting, sculpture, music, drama, book making, or other multimedia arts processes. In a structured session, there is a reflection on a specific topic or theme before the art making begins (or gentle guidance of the art-making process that allows for individual interpretation of the guidance) and in an open session there is no reflection or guidance, just open access to the specific art form of that session to be done individually or in groups, however the participants would like to engage with the art modality.

Sharing circles include a process of inviting participants to sit in a circle and share their artwork, either visually or verbally or both, after the art-making process is complete. This process promotes the normalization of feelings and emotions, supports the development of empathy, and creates a mechanism through which participants gain an increased understanding of themselves and each other, strengthening group bonding and a supportive group atmosphere.

Grounding activities include short activities intended to reflect on the experience of the session, focus on positive future orientation, and close the session together with a common action or reflection. Examples include a quick round of verbal reflection on how everyone is feeling, a fun energizer, a group song or dance, or a reflection on what participants are looking forward to later that day or week. Relaxation activities can also be used for grounding at the end of a session.

Goals of the HEART Program

The combination of activities in each session, done on weekly basis, over many months (often following the school year) creates a consistent, reliable, and emotionally supportive environment where children can support themselves and each other to process and recover from stress and to develop skills to support future stress processing and recovery.

The program is intentionally designed to include a variety of different types of activities using different art forms and a variety of logistical methods for engaging with those activities and related art forms. For example, some art-making processes are done individually and some are done in pairs or small groups. This approach allows for a variety of experiences including individual and group decision making, individual self-expression and group communication, individual and group coordination, individual and group problem solving, and many other processes that promote individual and group well-being while enhancing development and learning.

The topics of the structured sessions are intended to promote improved understanding of feelings, emotions and stress reactions, communication of ideas and experiences, identification of individual and group strengths and resources, and a promotion of a positive future orientation. The sessions are adjusted, in both content and logistical process, to the age of the participants. Thus, the way the program is delivered to the 4–7 age group differs from that for the 8–12 age group and the 13–18 age group, and the way the program is delivered to adults varies from the way it is delivered to children and youth.

HEART was intentionally designed to include multiple art forms including painting, drawing, sculpture, music, dance, drama, book making, and others. This design is partly to provide a diversity of activities that will appeal to more children (some will prefer certain art forms to others) and partly to ensure that engaging in HEART over time will be more likely to have diverse positive neurological impacts because each art form relates to different sensory stimuli that correlate to different lobes of the brain that are responsible for stress processing and recovery, development, and learning. The neuroscience of the expressive arts is discussed in more detail in later chapters.

In the second half of this book, specifically in Chapters 4 to 10, the specifics of the HEART program are explored in more detail, including the experience of using the program to support different age groups, adapting the program to different contexts, and customizing the program to support specific populations affected by different types of adversities. It also explores the logistics of the global program including financing, management, stakeholder partnerships, challenges, successes, and future goals. But before the program can be explored in more detail, we first need to discuss the theory, research, and evidence that informs the design of the HEART program and its goal of supporting the psychosocial well-being of children and adults affected by adversity.

Notes

1   The experts who collaboratively contributed to the design, piloting, review, revision, and standardization of the HEART program originate from eight different countries in Asia, the Middle East, Africa, and North America.

2   In situations in which a school does not have dedicated time or space for weekly HEART sessions during the regular school day, the program can be organized as an after-school activity. In some cases, all children in the school can be accommodated. In other situations, there is a limit on how many can attend. In situations in which the program is limited, the school may decide to dedicate the program for a specific

grade level to ensure that all children have an opportunity to participate (assuming the program recurs for that grade level over many years so that all children in the school eventually pass through the grade level and thus through the HEART program).

3   The alternation schedule can vary. The most common variations include weekly alternations (structured one week and open the next) or monthly in which one open session is done per month while all other weeks in the month have structured sessions.

Chapter 2

Growing Through Adversity
Risks and Protective Factors for Children and Their Caregivers

Girija Kaimal, Rebekka Dieterich-Hartwell,
Bani Malhotra, Victoria Schwachter, and Asli Arslanbek

The Ecology of Childhood and Youth

Development in childhood and youth occurs across several dimensions, including physiological, social, emotional, cognitive, and artistic. Each of these areas typically involves developmental stages that lead to increased complexity and specialization in the children's abilities to respond to their environments. Along with the visible changes in their physical development, simultaneous changes occur in their inner lives. These include increasing awareness of their own emotional life and awareness of others around them in circles of interpersonal relationships. With each stage, they increasingly interact with and ideally become integral parts of larger swathes of society.

The idea that we as human beings are part of larger systems that connect individuals to society was defined as **ecological systems theory** (Bronfenbrenner, 2005). Bronfenbrenner (2005) characterized this theoretical perspective as evolving from the child's biologically influenced dispositions and his or her interactions with a diverse environment. The environment is understood as interrelated, nested structures composed of the **microsystem** (immediate relations between the child and the environment such as the family), the **mesosystem** (connections between and within the child's immediate settings such as the neighborhood, childcare center, or school), the **exosystem** (settings that may not contain children but affect them, such as their parents' workplaces, religious institutions, and community health services), the **macrosystem** (values, laws, customs, and culture), and the **chronosystem** (the ever-changing dynamic environment involving life changes and social issues) (Berk, 2019) (Figure 2.1).

This dynamic system recognizes the child's mind, body, physical world, and social world as a continuously organizing, integrated system that guides mastery of new skills (Berk, 2019). This development is a dynamic interplay between all these influences on a child. Development is thus not linear but rather a web of fibers branching out in many directions, each representing a different skill set that may undergo both continuous and stagewise transformations (Fischer & Bidell, 2006).

DOI: 10.4324/9781003367529-3

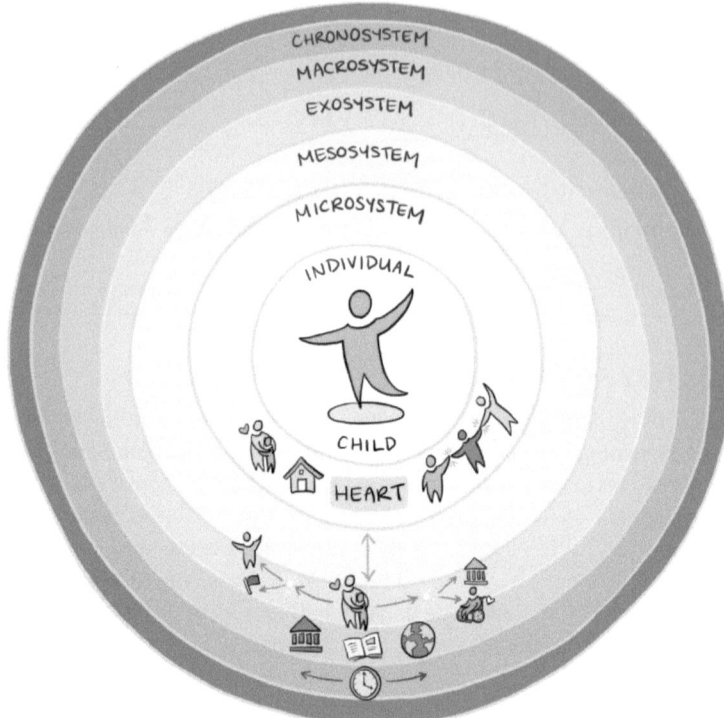

Figure 2.1 Social Ecological Framework for Development

Source: Kristyn S. Stickley

Children of all ages and of differing abilities navigate the processes of growing differently. Moreover, child development and human functioning are deeply embedded in nested contexts. The idea that children grow in interdependent contexts of family and community informs HEART and its work around the world. HEART implements its program within the contextual influences on a child and views the child's development within a complex system of relationships with the surrounding environment.

Eustress, Distress, and the Context of the Developing Child

For all children, as they develop, some amount of stress is expected and needed for healthy growth: This stress is referred to as **eustress** (Selye, 1951). Eustress helps optimize performance and develop strength and skills. Navigating routine new experiences and challenges that a child encounters helps build mastery and skill. For a developing child, eustress might comprise experiences such as falling and getting up repeatedly to learning to use the body, arms, legs, and fingers to master gross and fine motor control. Similarly, it includes navigating social interactions, learning to name and recognize feelings and emotions, and mastering self-regulation and self-expression. The struggle to master developmental milestones, to learn about the world, and to understand the people and things in it, differentiating between safe and unsafe places where one might thrive and where one might not, is the work of childhood and youth. Eustress then is a catalyst: a challenge that helps us level up and develop.

Beyond a point though, stress in any aspect of a child's life, including the effects of the community and of distress in the lives of the adults and family units, can become overwhelming and unmanageable. This type of stress changes from eustress to **distress**, which can be debilitating for the developing child. The body and mind of a developing child are vulnerable to excessive challenges and distress because they shift the trajectory of the normative unfolding of developmental pathways. These include physical, emotional, and cognitive pathways. Chronic distress from adversities faced by children and families can have lifelong impacts. These adverse childhood experiences (ACEs) have been associated with higher risks of delayed development as well as with physical and mental illnesses later in life. Adversity does not, however, have to be fixed in its outcomes. The human brain is deeply adaptive, and negative impacts can be offset with protective experiences including nurturing adults, stable educational experiences, and creative expressive opportunities. In the following sections, we summarize the current state of knowledge about the impacts of adverse experiences as well as how they can be mitigated with known protective factors.

Adverse Childhood Experiences

What are adverse childhood experiences or ACEs and why are they relevant to children and the adults in their communities? **ACEs** (CDC, 2023b) are extremely stressful or potentially traumatic events that occur in childhood and youth. ACEs can take place at the individual, familial, or community level. They can include experiencing violence, abuse, or neglect; witnessing violence in the home or community; and experiencing the unexpected deaths of friends or family members. The environment that undermines a child's sense of safety is also considered an ACE. An ACE can include but is not limited to substance abuse; mental health challenges; instability due to parental absence, loss, or separation; unstable housing and discrimination; and food insecurity. Some estimates place almost 50% of the population worldwide as having experienced one or more ACEs (Touloumakos & Barrable, 2020).

ACEs have been tracked across the world. It is estimated that 535 million children—about one in four of the world's children—live in countries affected by ACEs due to natural or man-made hazards. Moreover, children also account for over half of the displaced people and refugee groups around the world (UNICEF 2016, 2017). Humanitarian emergencies affect children in complex ways, including the increased risks of multiple co-occurring health challenges such as mental illnesses, acute or chronic malnutrition, infectious diseases, and inconsistent health care (Kohrt & Carruth, 2020). Living in emergency settings like war zones can increase the risk of traumatic brain injury; nerve and physical injuries that become chronic conditions due to disrupted care; preventable diseases like polio and measles; and even increased vulnerability to chronic health conditions (Mateen, 2010).

Experiences like abuse, lack of resources, neglect, caregiver losses, and violence have been related to risky behaviors, chronic health conditions, and even early death (Anda et al., 2010). It can be assumed that multiple health challenges co-occur and that the differences vary based on the child's sociocultural context. A meta-analysis that synthesized research (206 studies from 22 countries) on ACEs around the world over the past 25 years found that children from families that faced four or more ACEs were more likely to experience challenges in adulthood including mental health issues, substance misuse, homelessness, and poverty (Madigan et al., 2023). Similarly, food insecurities in their developmental history affected children's health outcomes including anxiety and an increased risk of diabetes. Recognizing the interplay of family history and community context is therefore essential to provide interventions that can offset these multiple challenges (Holz et al., 2023).

These difficult experiences in the developing years of childhood and youth can impact brain wiring and physiological and psychological health across the lifespan (Luby et al., 2013) in ways that are still being studied. For example, harsh and abusive parenting behaviors have been found to have lifelong effects on brain volume, fear response, and connectivity in the brain (Suffren et al., 2021). Childhood adversities increase the risk of mental and physical ill health in adulthood such as post-traumatic stress disorder (PTSD), substance use disorders, cardiovascular disease, weight-related disorders, mood disorders, and metabolic dysregulation disorders like diabetes. A review of brain imaging studies found evidence of significant changes in brain structures, as a result of childhood adversity and trauma. The findings that adversity affects the function and volume of key brain structures like the amygdala and hippocampus (Herzog & Schmahl, 2018) were salient.

For children who endure extreme distress, the amygdala (the part of the brain that assesses fear and threats) becomes dysregulated and either overreacts or becomes numb to external perceptions of threat and danger. This dysregulation affects a developing child's understanding and ability to determine what is safe and unsafe in the world. A real-life consequence then becomes that the child makes maladaptive choices because their perception of an external threat is inaccurate and what might be unsafe is perceived as safe because it is familiar.

The hippocampus, which is associated with memory processing, is another structure affected by trauma and adversity that affects the developing child's ability to retain and learn from experiences.

In addition to the impact of adversities across the childhood years, brain development occurs in spurts during early childhood and then again in the early preteen years, which are sensitive time periods that impact development in significant ways. For example, the ages of 10 to 11 years have been found to be particularly sensitive to amygdala development, with lifelong negative impacts when children experienced abuse at these ages (Teicher & Parriger, 2015). When children witness violence (including domestic violence) in this sensitive period of brain development and neural pruning, they are at risk of reduced cortical development and visual sensitivity later in life (Tomoda et al., 2012).) Similarly, older children facing multiple stressors had significantly more symptoms of post-traumatic stress compared with those who had faced fewer stressors (Dubow et al., 2012). The stress of living in conditions of communal violence and trauma or of more personal challenges, such as disability and poverty, can have effects that compound exponentially over time. Poverty and a lack of nurturing resources in the environment in childhood have been found to impact brain development, including reduction in gray matter and reduced volume in the frontal and temporal lobes and the hippocampus (Hair et al., 2015) as well as reduced brain volume. These reductions can have significant impacts on functioning and including maladaptive response pathways and behaviors. (Hackman & Farah, 2009; Hair et al., 2015; Luby et al., 2013; Noble et al., 2015)

In particular, it is worth noting that as children develop, they gain a refined and nuanced understanding of emotions. According to Kandel (2012), our primal instincts are **approach** and **avoidance**. At a very basic level our responses to the world around us is to approach things that interest us and avoid things that we perceive as harmful. As our brains and bodies mature, we develop words and meanings associated with these two instincts and identify the specific feelings and emotions associated with different emotional experiences and people. To know and to be able to name these feelings and emotions accurately or at least as well as we can, become essential to our ability to better integrate them into our life stories and our ongoing life narratives. Children living in the stress of poverty have more difficulty understanding and coping with emotions, which in turn can affect later social and academic milestones (Izard et al., 2008). Emotional regulation and the capacity to process difficult emotions are affected when the developing child experiences constant threats and stresses. It is important to note that most theories and research are framed around typically developing children and that models of human development often leave out people with disabilities, leading to rigid and exclusive perceptions about what it means to be an adult (Jordan & Tseris, 2017). Brain development is inherently linked with disability, because the multidimensionality of human functioning

> reflects the interactive nature of disability and the significant role that personal and contextual factors play in the expression of genes and brain development. There is a dynamic and reciprocal engagement between intellectual functioning, adaptive behavior, health, one's context and participation, and the size and complexity of the discrepancy between personal competence and environmental demands.
>
> (Schalock et al., 2019)

As discussed previously, the results of the research on the neurobiological impacts of adversities are compelling and unequivocal. If these experiences remain unaddressed, significant lifelong adverse consequences can result. The research on these outcomes highlights the risks and the need for and impact of early interventions in the growing years.

What then are ways to counter the impacts of life adversities on the developing child? There is hope because the human brain is adaptable. This adaptability is referred to as **neuroplasticity**. Neuroplasticity is the idea that the neural connections and pathways in the brain can be modified and updated with new experiences. Neural pathways can be altered to better serve us and help us make choices that enhance survival and thriving. The earlier these opportunities for rewiring that exist for a child, facing adversities especially during sensitive periods of development, the better are the potential outcomes across the life span.

Protective and Compensatory Experiences

Adversities in life may be unavoidable, but there are ways to counter the negative impacts of these challenges. These are referred to as **protective and compensatory experiences** (PACES) or benevolent childhood experiences (Narayan et al., 2018): experiences that offset the negative impacts of adversities and make them manageable or help reduce the damage they might cause. PACES (Hays-Grudo & Morris, 2020) include protective experiences such as supportive relationships, productive activities, and mind-sets of learning from adverse experiences. These can include having unconditional love from a parent/caregiver or teacher; having a best friend; being part of a social group; having support from an adult outside of the family; living in a clean, safe home with enough food; having resources and opportunities to learn; engaging in a hobby; engaging in regular physical activity; having predictable daily routines and fair rules; and having opportunities to have a positive self-concept, feelings, and beliefs. Access to nature and the natural environment is also found to be protective (Toulomakos & Barrable, 2020).

These benevolent experiences have been found to offset the effects of difficult times (Narayan et al., 2018), including those engendered by the recent COVID-19 pandemic. The benevolent experiences resulted in lowered stress, depression, and loneliness among children who were otherwise considered living in adversity (Doom et al., 2021). Emotional support interventions in the form of enhanced cognitive stimulation, support, and nurturance applied during the preschool period of development have powerful positive effects on adult outcomes. There is evidence that the earlier we offer enriched opportunities (e.g., during the preschool period) to remedy the early negative environmental stresses, the better are the outcomes compared with similar interventions applied in later childhood, adolescence, and early adulthood (Heckman et al., 2006).

Creating a Nurturing Environment

"Every child deserves a champion—an adult who will never give up on them, who understands the power of connection and insists that they become the best that they can possibly be" (Pierson, 2013). As discussed previously, adverse experiences can have lifelong negative health impacts but can be offset with protective experiences, primarily the presence of nurturing adults who believe in and love the child unconditionally. The role of a mentally and physically healthy adult in a child's life is deeply intertwined with the child's well-being and is a key protective factor. The child development scholar, Masten (2014), referred to these elements as **ordinary magic**: the simple everyday things like the love and support of a caring adult that help children and youth develop the strength to live and love well. These factors can help children manage their emotions, self-regulate, understand their experiences, gain self-confidence, and feel safe in the face of overwhelming external threats to well-being.

Parenting, Caregiving, Attachment, and Well-Being

The effect of early relationship attachments (of children with caregivers) on cognitive and emotional capacities has been widely studied. The infant's emotional tie to the caregiver is an evolved response that promotes survival (Berk, 2019). As children depend fully on their caregivers for survival, they form an internal working model or expectations about attachment figures and their availability of support during times of stress (Bowlby, 1980). As a result of these early experiences, children form either secure or insecure attachments. Secure attachments occur when the caregiver is consistent and loving and offers the child a view of the world as a safe place where other humans can be trusted. Insecure attachments result when the caregivers are neglectful, abusive, and/or inconsistent. Positive supportive relationships can offset early insecure attachments including those with peers and later those with partners and one's own children.

In many societies and cultures around the world, children are not reared solely by parents or mothers alone but are enmeshed in communities and larger groups and are brought up in a model of multiple caregiving that affects their emotional and cognitive understanding of social relationships (Seymour, 2013). These may take the form of focused, or person-specific attachment, or diffused attachment, where acknowledgment of security for a child might be diffused among different individuals (Meehan & Hawks, 2013). Such availability and presence of multiple adults may in turn help produce interpersonal trust and interdependence (Seymour, 2013). Wadende, Morara, and Oburu (2016) assert that child development is deeply embedded in their community with education in the mental, physical, emotional, and social aspects as preparation for life. The authors suggest that community participation in offering children opportunities to engage in practical, productive, and responsible livelihood activities prepares them for success in transitions including that from home to formal schooling.

Extensive cross-cultural research confirms the basic principles of attachment theory, including secure attachment and insecure attachment with three subcategories—avoidant, ambivalent, and disorganized (Mesman, van Ijzendoorn, & Sagi-Schwartz, 2016), but finds that ways of expressing attachment and exploration vary, depending on local customs, cultural norms, and economic resources. Secure attachment to caregivers sets the child up for a lifetime of relationship expectations and dynamics. Different parenting styles have shown to affect attachment, child development, and well-being. When the caregiving environment is inconsistent or neglectful, children form insecure attachments. These insecure attachment styles can be anxious, avoidant, or fearful (Ainsworth et al., 1978; Berk, 2019; Main & Solomon, 1990). **Anxious attachment** is a response to intrusive or alternately caring and harsh parenting. Children living with this type of attachment style become fearful of abandonment and sensitive to changes in the moods of their caregivers and the environment. **Avoidant attachments** are a response to neglect and abandonment such that the child internalizes early that there will be nobody available to them when they need care and nurturance. As such, they teach themselves to be self-sufficient and self-reliant and avoid close relationships for fear of loss of independence and autonomy (stemming from a deep fear of intimate relationships as being unsafe and unfamiliar). Last, **fearful or disorganized attachment** arises from profoundly abusive early childhood contexts where the child is unable to form any stable sense of relationships with caregivers or peers. This internal working model of relationships and attachment to others becomes a core part of a child's personality, serving as a guide for future relationships (Greenberg, Cicchetti, & Cummings, 1990). It is essential to note here that there are differences in context when considering parenting and attachment styles (Brown,

Hawkins-Rodgers, & Kapadia, 2008), and most importantly insecure attachment styles can move more to the secure type when given the opportunity for
safety, authenticity, and belonging.

The beauty of the neural processes in the brain is that they respond to both
positive and negative stimuli from the environment. Thus, the brain adapts
behaviors and responses based on traumatic events but also to restorative and
nurturing events. The human brain, being adaptable, allows the developing child
to form new and nurturing interpersonal relationships with adults when these are
available, including other caregivers and adults in the community. Psychologist
Lev Vygotsky emphasized that language and cultural context in children's lives
paved the way for research on development across cultures, ethnic groups, and
specific environmental conditions. His **sociocultural theory** "focuses on how
culture—the values, beliefs, customs, and skills of a social group—is transmitted to the next generation" (Berk, 2015). Vygotsky recognized **sign systems** or **cultural semiotic systems** that allowed symbolic representation of
knowledge through drawing pictures, reading, writing, maps, and diagrams
(Goswami, 2008). The availability of these cultural tools through social interaction between children and more knowledgeable members of society (adults,
teachers) mediated children's development across cultural settings. Vygotsky's
concept of **zone of proximal development**—the difference between what children can do alone and what they can do under collaboration with and guidance
from peers/adults—has been a critical contribution to the education of children
in school settings (Goswami, 2008).

Unlike many of his predecessors and contemporaries, Vygotsky studied the
development of children with disabilities. He conceptualized disability not as
a biological condition but as the social consequence of a biological condition
(Kozulin & Gindis, 2007). He therefore not only recognized that there are differences in individuals' development but that such differences come from a
combination of natural and cultural causes (Vik & Somby, 2018). Vygotsky, in
particular, emphasized the importance of play as crucial to psychological functioning and child development in facilitating self-regulation, abstract thinking,
and imagination (Vygotsky, 1978) that provided a "critical bridge between per-
ceptual/situational constraints of early childhood, and adult thought" (Goswami,
2008). For children with disabilities, their attachment style may be further
influenced by frequent separation from their caregivers or by stressed parents
resorting to "pathological parenting" (Frankish, 2018). The parents and caregivers also need nurturance so that they can provide a supportive developmental
environment for the child (CDC, 2023a). In particular, parents and caregivers of
children with special needs need support around childrearing strategies, understanding differences in developmental trajectories, managing own distress and
sense of community and belonging (Heiman, 2021).

Sustaining a Nurturing Environment: Impact on Caregivers at Home and School and in the Community

For all humans, but particularly for children, play and creativity are both associated with safety and thus serve as an antidote to stress. To be able to play without any demands of a specific outcome is essential for exploration and to develop the ability to problem solve in creative ways. For example, having access to natural settings has been associated with lower cortisol levels (Touloumakos & Barrable, 2020): Children aged 9–10 who had had access to outdoor environments had steadier diurnal cortisol levels later in life (Dettweiler et al., 2017). Adaptive capacity for self-regulation was found to be higher for kindergarten children who had access to playgrounds (Taylor & Butts-Wilmsmeyer, 2020). Children also learn faster with play. One study indicated that children learned faster through play compared with adults because of the neurotransmitter gamma aminobutyric acid (GABA) (Frank et al., 2022). GABA is an inhibitory neurotransmitter that helps process and integrate learning in adults. It exists in lower levels in children, which allows for rapid learning even if it is associated with lower impulse control.

Playful environments that are not as restrictive thus potentially create a rapid learning environment for children. Playfulness is associated with safety; as such, all learning and exploration that occur in safe spaces lower stress levels and allow for deeper engagement, less fear of making mistakes, and less defined patterns and ways of being. In adults, GABA works to reduce neuronal activity; consequently, it helps with rest, sleep, and reducing stress. When children face excessive stress in childhood, their levels of GABA are imbalanced in adulthood and are often lower than average, which affects a range of mood and relaxation functions (Hepsomali et al., 2023). More information on the protective roles of creativity and play is provided in Chapter 3.

Because a child is learning to navigate the world, everyone and everything around them offer them lessons on how to live, how to be, and how to navigate challenges. Children learn how to see themselves in the world through these early experiences. They are thus profoundly shaped by those around them every day including family members, community members, and peers as well as by interactions with formal and informal caregivers. Families of origin are often the first community for children, and much of their worldview is shaped forever by these early experiences, including attachment styles, future relationships, and life choices. The protective role of attachment and of belonging to a community is particularly salient for children and adults in navigating these challenges.

Economic Adversities and Relationships with Parents and Caregivers

To be faced with adversity such as life-threatening trauma or chronic stress can be demanding on any relationship. Adults become anxious and fearful and children in turn sense this danger and imminent threats to their safety and belonging. To sustain unwavering love and mutual respect among adults and unconditional positive regard and nurturance to children then is a protective factor. To have a secure attachment relationship is a shield and armor to any child and to every adult. Adversities that affect a child can reasonably be expected to affect adults as well, and supporting the adults ensures that they can be effective in their caregiving responsibilities.

What then are the unique needs of adults in a child's life—adults with needs and struggles of their own? To be faced with chronic stressors of resources, violence, poverty, and similar challenges can affect adults and deplete their ability to be compassionate caregivers and educators. These factors occur on top of ongoing parental and caregiving stresses, which can vary across family situations, but are typically found to be significant in families of children with disabilities (Nurullah, 2013). Facing and viewing persistent humanitarian and community difficulties result in vicarious trauma and compassion fatigue for youth and adults in any community. Staff and workers in settings of chronic stress and trauma might face additional difficulties of operational challenges, limited resources, and fatigue of having no respite far from home. Supporting children then necessarily involves supporting adults and caregivers in the community.

Families who live below the poverty line encounter enormous stressors including financial challenges and material deprivations. In addition, poverty is frequently accompanied by other chronic circumstances such as neighborhood violence and discrimination that diminish family members' well-being and trigger traumatic stress (Slopen et al., 2016). Numerous studies have detailed the relationship between family poverty and children's development. For example, it has been shown that preschool children from low-income families have significantly more behavioral problems than other children in that age group (Holtz, Fox, & Meurer, 2015). A recent mixed methods study (Ho et al., 2022) found that the wide range of difficulties associated with poverty increased the tendency for caregivers to turn to harsh parenting practices that negatively affected their relationships with their children. More specifically, poverty affected the perceptions of the caregiver role, including feelings of being overwhelmed; long working hours and material deprivations compromised the caregiver–child connection; social networks were hard to come by due to barriers created by poverty; and caregiver adults reported feeling shame, which prevented them from seeking support.

Impacts of Adversities on Care Workers

In addition to parents and caregivers, adults in the helping professions are exposed to significant trauma or chronic stress, including exposure to human suffering such as war, poverty, abuse, and natural disasters. There are many ways in which exposure can impact functioning, including secondary stress, vicarious trauma, compassion fatigue, and burnout. When care workers witness the suffering of children in their care, they can experience what is referred to as vicarious trauma (van Dernoot Lipsky & Burk, 2009). According to van Dernoot Lipsky & Burk (2009), this vicarious trauma or trauma exposure response refers to the transformation that takes place within us as a result of exposure to the suffering of other living beings. Since human beings are naturally wired for understanding and being responsive to the pain of others, vicarious trauma emerges from our empathic engagement with the traumatic experiences of those around us (Pearlman & Saakvitne, 1995). Vicarious trauma can be observed through feelings of hopelessness and helplessness, the sense that one can never do enough, hypervigilance, difficulty embracing complexity, minimizing the suffering one is exposed to, chronic exhaustion and physical illness, avoidance and difficulty listening, feelings of numbness and challenges empathizing with others, addictions, and inaccurately perceiving the grandiosity to one's work (Branson, 2019, van Dernoot Lipsky & Burk, 2009). Similarly to vicarious trauma is **Secondary Traumatic Stress** (STS) which refers to behaviors and emotions resulting from knowledge about a traumatizing event experienced by a significant other. It is the stress resulting from helping or wanting to help a traumatized or suffering person that is emotionally connected to us in meaningful ways (Figley, 1999). STS is commonly used for professionals (family, friends, and human services personnel) who encounter people who experience trauma but who do not develop an ongoing empathic relationship with the trauma survivors (Branson, 2019).

Similarly, **compassion fatigue** can develop in response to caring for people in significant emotional pain and physical distress (Figley, 1995). Compassion fatigue is an overall dysfunction and exhaustion of biological, psychological, and social well-being related to overwhelming caregiving demands. According to Matthieu (2007), some of the characteristics of compassion fatigue are exhaustion, anger, and irritability. Negative coping behaviors could include self-medication (e.g., excessive alcohol and drug use) alongside the reduced ability to feel sympathy and empathy, a diminished sense of enjoyment or satisfaction with work, increased absenteeism, and an impaired ability to make decisions and care for dependent others. In essence, it is a change in the empathic capacity of a caregiver due to the prolonged and overwhelming stress of caregiving (Lynch a& Lobo, 2012). These effects obviously can impact standards of care and relationships with colleagues and can sometimes lead to more serious mental health conditions such as PTSD, anxiety, or depression.

In addition to the stressors associated with knowing individuals who have experienced trauma, humanitarian workers also navigate stressors related their work. These include **operational** and **organizational stressors** (Jachens, 2019). Operational stressors are types of stressors inherent in the type of humanitarian aid work, such as working long hours, exposure to adversities active in the setting, and working and living in a stressful environment. Organizational stressors are stressors related to a particular humanitarian aid organization. These can include stressors related to workload, lack of support from line managers and senior management, poor team dynamics, discrimination, lack of accommodations for disability, or a toxic working culture (Jachens, 2019). Research focused on these issues underscores high rates of negative mental and physical health outcomes for aid workers. Chief among these is **burnout** which is a condition that develops gradually and can lead to emotional exhaustion and a sense of reduced personal accomplishment that can occur among individuals who work with people in chronic and/or acute distress (Maslach, Jackson, & Leiter, 1996).

There are several ways to address the psychological well-being of humanitarian workers. Efforts can be made pre-emptively to support individuals working in such emotionally and physically demanding environments. Making available appropriate guidelines/handbooks; providing effective training in supporting other team members; making available ongoing support groups for debriefing of emotional responses; balancing direct client work with activities that enhance hope and empowerment with community engagement and collaborations; and providing interventions aimed at improving psychological skills and positive coping strategies (Bell, Shanti, & Dalton, 2003;Office of Victims of Crime, n.d; Bardach et al., 2022).

Post-Traumatic Growth, Resilience, and Antidotes to Distress

There is much research about post-traumatic stress and the lifelong impacts of adverse events. Our capacity to cope and to respond to the most adverse of situations is a point of hope and a testament to the abiding adaptability and creativity of the human spirit. These include learning and growing from intensely challenging experiences as well as recognizing the human capacity to recreate and adapt. We have all known people who have taken adversity and transformed it into a life purpose and mission. Tedeschi and Calhoun (1996) named this concept Post-Traumatic Growth (PTG). PTG refers to positive psychological changes that some people have after experiencing a traumatic event that leads to a new way of life by building on existing and newly identified strengths. It is not the same as **resilience**, because resilience refers to returning to how things were: being able to bounce back from challenges. Tedeschi and Calhoun (1996) asserted that, unlike resilience, PTG is about being transformed by the adverse experience into a newer self that is different and is operating at a completely different level than before. It is a manifestation of our inherent adaptability, strengths, and assets as human beings.

Taleb (2014) coined a similar term, **antifragility**, which is the capacity to become strengthened rather than defeated by adversity. **Fragility** is the likelihood of breaking easily. Antifragility as the ability to be strengthened by adversity, not just the ability to resist challenges and difficulties. It is similar to the idea of eustress (small doses of challenges that strengthen us) versus distress, which are challenges that are painful and debilitating (Selye, 1951). Similar to the idea of eustress and distress, children and adults are strengthened in ways that make distress manageable. Exercise essentially breaks down muscles and rebuilds them stronger. Vaccinations work on the same principle. Small doses of an agent that causes an illness can lead to an immune response. The difficulty of course is when the challenges are life-threatening beyond one's capacity to deal with them. Having tools, awareness, and strategies help us cope and respond with antifragility and seek PTG. The transformations might be spiritual, personal physical strengths, new appreciation for life, new purpose, new focus and possibilities, none of which would have been conceivable prior to the traumatic experience. Processing the traumatic experiences in a safe, creative, and supportive context can lead us to have new perspectives, self-awareness, interpersonal awareness, an understanding of how to manage triggers, a compassionate stance toward self and others, and a self that is shaped and defined by the experiences that could have and perhaps did lead to post-traumatic stress but also led to transformation and growth.

PTG is not to be confused with **toxic positivity**, which forces platitudes and simplistic tropes, or about minimizing grief and loss. PTG is instead about awareness and reconciliation that arose from an intensely painful period in one's life. It is likely that there are predisposing traits that affect our capacity for PTG. Dunn et al. (2014) found that, in Hurricane Katrina survivors, variants in the gene RGS2 significantly interacted with levels of exposure to the hurricane to predict PTG. RGS2 is linked to fear-related disorders, such as PTSD, panic disorder, and anxiety. The authors do propose caution in attributing all PTG to genetics, because so much of our adult self is defined by developmental experiences and not necessarily by genetic predispositions alone.

Key Takeaways

Human development in childhood and youth is a complex interplay of interactions with the family and the community. These interactions impact several dimensions of growth including physiological, socioemotional, relational, cognitive, and artistic development. Play and creativity are integral to the healthy development of the inner and social lives of children: Nurturing these activities allows children to know life as a space to thrive. Adverse childhood experiences can have lifelong impacts on physical and emotional health. Adults in the lives of children, including family members, teachers, caregivers, and others they know and learn from in the community, are impacted by the same challenges and adversities experienced by the children. Their responses can have detrimental impacts; however, there are several established ways to counter these impacts, including working with creative and community resources. These topics are discussed further in Chapter 3.

Chapter 3

Creative Resources

How the Expressive Arts Help Children and Adults Develop and Cope with Adversities

Girija Kaimal, Rebekka Dieterich-Hartwell, Bani Malhotra, Victoria Schwachter, Asli Arslanbek, and Kristyn S. Stickley

Universality and Access to Artistic and Creative Practices for Psychosocial Well-being

The mental health and psychosocial support needs of the world far outweigh the availability of clinicians and mental health workers that can provide them. According to the World Health Organization, **mental health** is defined as a state of well-being in which a person realizes their abilities, can respond effectively with the normal stresses of life, can work productively, and is able to make a contribution to their community (WHO, 2022). Mental health disorders are a cause of disability for one in six people globally. According to the World Health Organization's World Mental Health Report, at present most human psychosocial needs have gone undetected and unserved, even though it is anticipated that one in three adults will need mental health care in their lifetimes. These unaddressed mental health needs have public health, socioeconomic, and human rights costs. The stigma around mental health and psychosocial well-being is a significant barrier as well, which both prevents access to care and the availability of care. Given the global challenges in the mental health-care workforce (half the world averages one psychiatrist per country) (WHO, 2022), the need to provide psychosocial support that is scalable and accessible is an urgent imperative. Offering psychosocial competencies that are locally adapted and community-led can result in preventive interventions to promote mental health and psychosocial well-being.

Although not widely known, arts-based psychosocial support is an increasingly effective way to offer accessible and scalable psychosocial support to individuals and communities in need. What then are the unique and sustainable contributions of arts-based psychosocial support compared with those of other mental health support programs offered to communities living in adversity?

The idea that engaging in expressive arts activities promotes psychosocial well-being in addition to promoting prosocial development is not new. Historically, artistic and creative expressive forms have emerged spontaneously in all communities around the world. To be a creative problem solver is a unique

DOI: 10.4324/9781003367529-4

attribute of being human and is directly related to how the human brain functions. The human brain is a predictive machine (Friston & Kiebel, 2009). It is constantly scanning the environment through its senses to assess threats and opportunities. In doing so, it creates future-based scenarios that enhance our chances of survival. It thus predicts what actions and behaviors will need to occur to ensure survival in the future. This exercise of imagining is ingrained in our ways of functioning and thinking. As a result, creative and artistic processes are natural ways to practice imagination, to enhance our problem-solving abilities, and most importantly to move beyond surviving to thriving.

Similarly, given this sequential or predictive thinking, the human brain is also wired to understand and align with storytelling that has a time orientation (past, present, and future) and cause-and-effect reasoning. Given that the brain is a predictive machine, we naturally understand sequential tales with a past, present, and future. We intuitively understand the sequencing of cause and effect and the characters that comprise a story. Every community around the world has such stories in the forms of myths and local legends. Levi-Strauss (1950) referred to this in identifying commonalities in community stories. He referred to mythological tales from around the world as the original forms of therapy because they provided us with symbolic representations of struggles and the ways in which imaginary humans have responded to and overcome them.

Every community around the world has spontaneously developed their own unique artistic practices, creative resources, stories, and metaphors. These indigenous practices have the arts embedded in everyday life including in the crafting of objects used for everyday activities, integration of arts music and dance in rituals and celebrations, and use of natural media and materials from the natural resources of the region (Nagarajan, 2018). The creative and artistic practices serve to both celebrate joyous occasions and to cope with distress and adversity (Kaimal, 2022; Menakem, 2017). Embedded in these arts practices are the rewarding feelings of joy that come from making objects of everyday living and the social connected and well-being including intergenerational exchanges through the act of creative self-expression together, creating. Most indigenous arts practices have simple elements that can be combined to create complex compositions (Arslanbek, Malhotra, and Kaimal, 2022; Kaimal, 2022). These everyday arts practices are inclusive of the members of the community and help in promoting resilience and the regulation of emotions.

Creative thinking, imagination, and artistic expression are natural and innate aspects of a child's development and human functioning. To be able to imagine, to play, to create, and to tell stories are manifestations of how our brains work. In trying to predict the future, in order to survive, we have also naturally developed this gift of artistic expression: creative expression that serves no purpose other than to bring joy and the satisfaction of making something (tangible or intangible). This creative resource or capacity that exists within all human beings, be they adults or children, can be particularly effective in times of stress and adversity. This capacity, when recognized and honed as a tool, can be a means to manage and move through challenges.

The Neuroscience of the Arts Including in Adversity

The inherent resilience and strength of creative tasks is supported by modern neuroscience research. The idea that physical effort helps us feel good has been demonstrated in the research conducted by neuroscientist Kelly Lambert (2008). She found that repetitive physical actions promote the production of serotonin, a neurochemical that reinforces a sense of joy and belonging. We are naturally creative as humans and meant to move to make, which helps us with a sense of confidence in overcoming challenges and helps us feel good. Being active, creative and expressive activates reward pathways in our brains, and helps us connect with ourselves and others in meaningful ways.

Recent research has greatly improved our knowledge of the neurological impact of making, viewing, and hearing creative works but still more remains to be understood. For example, there is compelling evidence that creative expression is a whole brain activity that integrates our sensory, perceptual, emotional, and cognitive functions (Limb & Braun, 2008; Kaimal et al., 2021). Engaging in expressive and creative activities are natural functions of the brain and also map on to aspects stress processing, learning, and development. There are multiple reward pathways in the brain that connect to different sensory systems. In particular, activities like movement and any type of efforts at "making" naturally activate reward pathways in our brain (Lambert, 2008). This is known as the effort-based reward system. For example, our sense of touch which is processed in the sensorimotor cortex and the parietal lobe of the brain is further enhanced when we do creative works of sculpting because the sensory system connects with the reward pathways, the emotional parts of the brain, and the prefrontal cortex that leads active decision making around the choices made by the sculptor. Just the simple act of sculpting (manipulating and feeling the clay in our hands) connects the sense of sight, smell, touch, and sound. The occipital lobe and temporal lobes which process sight and sound enable us to distinguish between colors, shapes, images, and sounds. The cerebellum, responsible for balance and physical coordination, connects to all physical activities, and in particular, to dance or other arts activities that involve physical movement (Bearss & deSouza, 2021; Cucca et al., 2018). The limbic system processes emotion and connects to the ideas behind the artistic expression, evoking memories and creating new associations. Last and most importantly for self-regulation, the frontal lobe is responsible for thinking functions and is involved in the process of every form of art making as individuals make decisions, organize their process, and

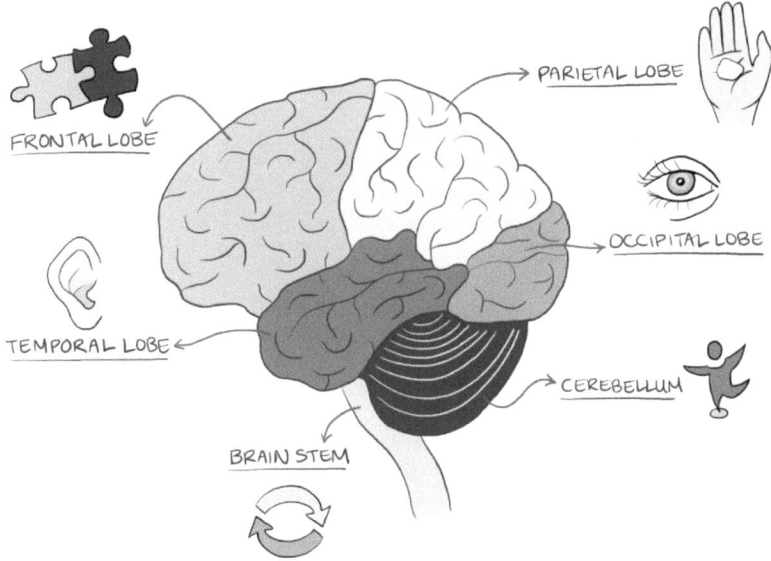

Figure 3.1 The Brain
Source: Kristyn S. Stickley

coordinate their interactions with others. To the brain, then, creative processes are a way to problem solve and keep our brains exercised and active for addressing the problems that will inevitably challenge us.

When we encounter acute or chronic stress, the brain perceives it as a threat and the primary emotion processing part of our brain (limbic system) takes over. As a result, the frontal lobe which is associated with logical and thoughtful decision making is less functional. In times of stressful events, the frontal lobe gets overridden by the limbic system, which is why during a stress response, we often feel as though we can't think clearly or make decisions. Engaging in arts activities can stimulate the frontal lobe and support sensory integration. Being able to coordinate and work with all our senses is particularly useful for individuals living and working in stressful conditions. Research has also demonstrated that stress hormones, such as cortisol, can reduce during periods of art making. Other changes such as reduced blood pressure and improved heart rate variability have also been seen as a result of engaging with the arts (Haiblum-Itskovitch et al., 2018; Mastandrea et al., 2018). Participating in the arts can improve the way different parts of the brain function and how they connect with each other (functional connectivity), including generating new neural pathways and strengthening ones that promote health.

To move, create, and be active is a natural instinct present in every child, see Table 3.1. Children play, dance, move, scribble, and sing as natural parts of

Table 3.1 Developmental Stages for Social, Emotional, Cognitive, and Artistic Development

Developmental stage	Visual arts	Music	Dance and movement	Cognition	Social and emotional development
Prenatal development (before birth)	Development of basic awareness of light	Exposure to sounds, vibrations, and pulse	In utero movement, including that in response to sounds	Subcortical structures develop	Response to prenatal stress and nutrition based on maternal context
Infancy and toddlerhood (ages 0–3 years)	Awareness of light, dark, and color; creating scribbles, awareness of shape and color, emerging motor skills	Forming sounds for expression and communication and emerging awareness of rhythms and melodies	Reflexes, gross motor movements including crawling, pulling up, and walking	Learning about the world and people through somato-sensory tools	Development of attachment styles with primary caregivers
Early childhood (ages 3–6 years)	Depiction of tadpole human figures with head and arms/feet; depiction of familiar objects	Increasing musical awareness including songs, increased accuracy of pitch, rhythm and musical engagement	Development of fine motor skills and increasing awareness of bodies in space and relative to others	Understanding interrelationships, categories, and roles of things in the world	Increasing autonomy and skill development
Middle and late childhood (ages 6–11 years)	Depiction of multiple people in context and environments development of perspective in drawings	Development of musical skills with instruments and voice. E.g., accurate reproduction of melodies, rhythms and group music making	Development of skills in full body movement and expression including intention and emotion	Ability to describe and categorize in concrete ways; emergence of ethical and moral thinking	Developing relationships with peers in addition to familial relationships

Preteen, adolescence (ages 11–18 years)	Efforts at realistic drawings and personalizing expressive styles	Development of self-definition and exploration in musical styles and preferences	Adapting to the developing body and its capacities through puberty	Understanding complexity, ambiguity, and the capacity for critical thinking	Developing individual preferences and identity and physical maturation
Youth and young adulthood (ages 18–25 years)	Choices to reject or stay connected with art, including receptive and/or expressive experiences	Choosing the role of music in life including receptive and/or expressive styles	Choosing the role of movement and dance in lifestyle and expressive choices	Developing individual choices and maturation in cognitive capacity	Developing identity in society and community; maturation of brain executive functioning

their development. Art making can help children at different levels, depending on their developmental phase. For example, art media and art processes help children explore kinesthetic and sensory perceptions. Touching cold clay, experiencing the rhythm of brush strokes, or dealing with the motor energy released through scribbling with crayons can all be included in the kinesthetic/sensory experience of working with art materials. The kinesthetic movements in art making can safely discharge energy to reduce bodily tension, or conversely, can stimulate the body as needed to increase sensory information processing (Hinz, 2009).

Creativity, Play, and Artistic Self-Expression as a Natural Part of Child Development

Art and play can help children develop an understanding of their emotions and help express and process them. Art and play allow children to channel their difficult emotions through materials, symbols, and metaphors. For instance, a child might tear, punch, poke, or pierce clay, making it a physically and emotionally safe alternative to absorb the anger the child might be experiencing (Rubin, 2012). This type of symbolic representations happens when the child mimics and relates to the art product or process (Rubin, 2012). Art making provides children with an opportunity to make sense of their emotions through expression, depiction, and symbolization of their emotional states (Shore, 2013). Symbolizing not only involves expression but also holds the possibility for articulating their self-narrative in a new and coherent way. By learning to express in the arts, children learn to connect the prefrontal cortex (executive parts of the brain) with the limbic (emotional) systems rather than respond reactively alone to distressing stimuli. This in turn helps with emotional awareness and self-regulation as they grow.

Development in the arts mirror neurotypical development in cognitive and socioemotional development in children and adults. In general, children's development unfolds over time to achieve increasing maturation in the physical, socioemotional, cognitive, and creative realms. Children mature at their own pace, and the stages do not necessarily follow specific age ranges (see Appendix 1 for a summary of basic developmental theories). These developmental milestones and developmental expectations also vary by culture and community.

As seen in Table 3.1, artistic development mirrors emotional, social, and cognitive development such that children steadily gain skills, mastery, and awareness. As children mature, much of the learning and development is intertwined with play. To be able to play is to be able to feel safe and explore without the negative consequences of failure. The opportunity for and the ability to play is thus a key part of healthy development in children.

The Role of Play in Coping, Learning, and Development

Play is a pivotal developmental act for children that allows them to conceptualize the world and determine how to orient themselves in it (Landreth, 2012). Explorative play also allows a child to make sense of uncertainties (Russ, 2016). Through play and exploration, children gain insights and solutions that are meaningful to them at their developmental level and that help them achieve the milestones they need to reach (Russ, 2016; Singha et al. 2020). Play that begins in childhood can be used to practice skills and strategies that lead to strengthening the creative learning muscle and to experience safety, exploration, and joy (Singha et al, 2020). As noted in Chapter 2, play is an integral part of development in children and youth. For children, play is learning and a space to actively practice efforts to master their challenges in an emotional world.

Mildred Parten was one of the first scholars to define our understanding of how children play at different ages. Parten (1932) posited a social theory of play that identified six stages children go through until they reach the age of 5: unoccupied, solitary, spectator, parallel, associative, and cooperative play. As seen in previous developmental stages, play also follows a trajectory that begins first by focusing on the self to then an increasing awareness of others (Table 3.2).

As seen in the Table 3.2, play is essential to social, emotional, and physical development in growing children. Play is also deeply connected with creativity in both children and adults. Shen (2023) defined play as a free behavior motivated by the interest or enjoyment inherent in the activity that is relatively

Table 3.2 Stage of Play in Early Childhood

Type of play	Age	Description
Unoccupied play	Prenatal to 3 months	Moving arms, legs, and body and discovering how they move
Solitary play	Birth to 2 years	Focusing on self and enjoying movements of own body limbs
Spectator play	2 years +	Enjoying observing others but not yet playing with them
Parallel play	2 years +	Playing and engaging in self-led activities in the presence of others without engaging with them
Associative play	2–4 years	Playing together in same activities without necessarily interacting
Cooperative play	4+ years	Playing with others in shared games and activities

free from external constraints. Playing can include object and language play, at work or during leisure, and is a way to explore imagination and is associated with enhanced creativity: The ability to become playful as needed helps a child to focus on the process rather than putting pressure on the outcome. Play manifests for both children and adults as safety in exploration and trying things out without the pressure of an outcome. Free, unstructured play in childhood, minimization of external constraints and a suspension of reality helps with play feeling like a psychologically free and safe space. Often this shows up with laughter and as humor as well. Humor can be defined as form of creative play in at all ages that is also considered creative and is associated with divergent thinking in adulthood (Russ & Wallace, 2013). Playfulness signifies safety for children and adults: a space to experience positive emotions and connection to self and others.

When adults feel unsafe, however, it affects their children's sense of play and safety as well. The loss of this playfulness can be detrimental to both the child and the family. Fearing for their child's safety, parents and caregivers can often become overprotective. This response is often justified in violent environments that necessitates inhibition of free play and exploration for children. This is a natural response for any caregivers to ensure the safety of the child and family unit.

It is possible however to support adult caregivers living in contexts of distress to create opportunities for safe and restorative developmentally restorative play. Teachers, for example, can support play in children by encouraging make-believe activities, pretend play, and guiding them in imaginative play scenarios (Bodrova, 2008). Encouraging children in playful exploration helps children stay flexible in their mindsets which in turn helps with lifelong creative problem solving and the ability to think through effectively in challenging situations. Teaching parents and children how to engage in learning-oriented, imaginative play games with children (Singer et al., 2003) was found to be particularly helpful for kindergarten children of parents from low socioeconomic status. Children whose parents and teachers support their naturally creative and imaginative lives have been found to show significant gains on an academic readiness assessment compared with those whose parents did not participate.

The interplay of the arts, creativity, play, and well-being are deeply intertwined in a child's development.

Arts-Based Interventions for Children and Youth Impacted by Adversities

Creative expression is inherent to human nature and nurturing that capacity in children provides them with inner resources for constructive and expressive problem solving throughout their lives. The arts are frequently a way to bring playfulness and a related sense of normalcy to otherwise challenging conditions for children and youth. This is because most educational systems around the world have classes for the arts and to be able to engage in arts experiences signal the safety and regular routines of education and school days. In times of distress and challenges, the arts can thus be a way for children to feel a sense of normalcy, to be able to voice, express, and communicate their worries and concerns in a nonverbal way (Kaimal et al., 2019; Snyder, Malhotra, & Kaimal, 2021). Taking into consideration that each of the different areas of the brain correlate to different sensory aspects of art making, art seeing, and art hearing, we can consider how the arts help support stress processing, learning, and development. When we create a safe and playful environment for self-expression, children can benefit from the arts by building neural connections and pathways that extend to aspects of academic learning. For example, the parietal lobe is involved in arithmetic processing and high-level mathematical thinking, both the frontal lobe and the cerebellum are involved in fine and gross motor skills, and the temporal lobe is involved in language processing, memory, and visual recognition as well as the processing of emotions.

Arts-based interventions that integrate free expression, learning, and play show promise for promoting psychosocial well-being. The intentional design of the HEART program to include multiple arts modalities such as drawing, painting, sculpting, drama, music, and dance, ensures that participants are exposed to different art forms on a regular basis over extended periods of time. Even within each individual HEART session, participants are exposed to different activities that promote a process of sensory integration by utilizing dramatic play and body movement (for short relaxation activities or energizers), a focused art making process (painting, sculpture, drawing, or other), and multiple processes of seeing colors, shapes, and images, as well as hearing music, speech, or other sounds. Thus, the diversity in arts offerings of the program not only ensures a broader range of activities that can appeal to more people but also ensures that those participating in the program have a diverse neurological benefit that comes from making art, seeing art, and hearing art within each individual session and over extended periods of time (often months or years). The approach of combining different art forms into holistic child support programming is echoed by the research of Nijs and Nicolaou (2021) who found music and movement-based activities as being particularly restorative for child refugees. They proposed that, by combining music and movement, children were able to engage in group connections and enjoy a sense of shared purpose, which in turn led to self-awareness, confidence, self-esteem, personal autonomy, connection, belonging, and bonding.

The arts and engaging in therapeutic and learning art activities with a facilitating adult can thus serve many psychosocial benefits, including expressing difficult or wordless emotions as well as gaining self-efficacy through the trials, errors, and successes of artistic and/or creative practice. Levick (1983) was one of the first art therapists to document and demonstrate how drawing was a nonverbal way for children to communicate. She referred to artistic expression as a means for communication and self-expression especially when children do not have words. Rubin (2005) further articulated the many ways in which we can support children who have faced adversities by offering a variety of art media and creating the safe and normalizing environment of a facilitating adult and peers in the art therapy studio.

It is important to note here that the creative arts therapies differ from arts-based programs. The creative and expressive arts therapies are mental health interventions provided by Master's-level-trained credentialed clinicians. These sessions are usually offered as psychotherapy by trained therapists with extensive supervised experiences within clinical settings. They have expertise in addressing psychological illnesses akin to psychologists, social workers, or other forms of professional mental health counseling. Arts-based psychosocial supports are inspired by these approaches but take a non-clinical stance focused on processing and reducing stress and improving psychosocial well-being. Given the limitations of trained providers worldwide, arts-based psychosocial supports allow for non-mental health professionals to bring the therapeutic values of creative and expressive experiences as public health interventions.

Studies have found that opportunities for engaging in the arts have profoundly positive impacts on verbal expression, reduce disruptive behaviors (Klorer & Robb, 2012), enhance academic achievement (Hardiman, Rinne, & Yarmolinskaya, 2014; Izard et al., 2008; Ruppert, 2006), and reduce stress (Brown et al., 2017), especially in students from socially and economically disadvantaged backgrounds. In a study of recreational arts engagement and mental well-being among youth in Australia, Davies et al. (2016) found that 100 hours or more of engagement in the arts in a year was associated with significantly higher levels of mental health and well-being compared with those who had fewer hours of arts engagement. Dance and music-based interventions for preschool children living in poverty also showed that children in arts-enriched environments (music and dance) demonstrated improved social skills, positive emotions, and fewer disruptive behaviors compared to children who did not participate in these programs (Lobo & Winsler, 2006; Brown & Sax, 2013). These benefits have been found to reach children across many contexts and experiences. For children with disabilities in particular, a 2020 scoping review of 12 health literature papers on arts programs found positive outcomes in regard to physical, cognitive, communication, social, emotional, or behavioral functioning in each of the studies (Edwards et al., 2020).

Dramatic play through theater arts is integral to children being able to practice and master their challenges and adversities (Wico, Huber, & Schnyder, 2021). It connects directly to pretend play as a way for children to navigate and try out ways to cope with difficulties. Pliske, Stauffer, and Werner-Lin (2021) highlighted how play promotes growth, particularly for children who have experienced ACEs. Play and the arts allow for identity formation through the integration of emotional and cognitive experiences as they relate to early adversities. Pretend play helps imagine scenarios and future self-regulation by practicing social and imaginative skills. Exploring and being able to navigate new terrain also gives the child the self-confidence needed to take risks that build skill and problem-solving techniques for the future. The therapeutic powers of play lie in the opportunity for self-expression, learning through metaphor (indirect tacit learning), emotional processing of experiences, for which we might not have words (things unsayable), managing stress, self-esteem, and creative problem solving. Play creates a context for self-expression, self-care, and positive emotions and a pathway to healing from adverse and distressing childhood experiences.

Performing arts experiences facilitated by a trained professional can be a way to bring children together in informal, playful, and creative ways. Monteiro and Wall (2011) highlighted the role of dance in particular, as being a conduit for individual and community healing. Dance and rituals link the body, mind, spirit, and history into integrative healing practices across the world. Dance and movement represent the body as a physical instrument and therefore a more effective nonverbal language for expressing needs, desires, and pain. Movement also is valued as a socially accepted way for self-expression, catharsis, altered physical and mental states, and transcendent spiritual connection to self and others.

Arts and creative expression are effective not only for children's development but can promote the psychosocial well-being of adults as well. Being able to express, play, and create freely in ways that are met with compassion and acceptance (without judgment on technique or skill) is a pathway to stress reduction and wellness for adults. Structured arts-based psychosocial support provides a mechanism whereby these opportunities are available to both children and adults.

Arts-Based Interventions to Support the Psychosocial Well-Being of Caregivers and Families

Improved psychosocial well-being of parents and caregivers has a direct and positive impact on children. Early childhood programs across the world have focused on promoting play to support both child and caregiver mental health (UNICEF, 2022). Examples of playful learning techniques, interactive activities, and educational games for caregivers and their children resulted in lower rates of depression in mothers and higher cognitive outcomes in children (UNICEF, 2022). An approach particular to caregivers is the use of the creative arts, including visual art, music, dance, and drama, to foster quality of life, agency, and self-efficacy. Even single sessions of visual arts-based interventions were found to reduce stress and improve mood among caregivers of patients facing chronic disease and hospice care (Kaimal, Mensinger, & Carroll-Haskins, 2020; Kaimal et al., 2022). Chapter 8 offers more specific examples of using the arts for parent and caregiver well-being through the experience of the HEART program.

Arts-Based Support for Staff Well-Being

Because of the severe lack of mental health professionals globally, offering accessible and scalable specialized creative arts therapies for staff in contexts of adversity is not feasible. Non-clinical arts-based psychosocial support that prioritizes the principles of therapeutic practice in an ethical way can be a viable alternative. Arts-based support for relief workers has demonstrated assistance for managing vicarious trauma and burnout from work (Bardot, 2018; Gavron et al., 2022; Ma & Penner, 2018), promoted empathy (Furlager, 2018) as well as helped identified strengths in local expressive traditions in the context of natural disasters (Huss et al., 2016, Gavron & Shemesh, 2022). Arts-based workshops (using visual arts and drama-based activities) have been found to help promote team cohesion and educate frontline humanitarian service providers with tools for self-care (Bardot, 2018). Arts-based workshops conducted for disaster management teams including collage tapestry, drawing, painting, reflective writing, meditation, sculpting, listening to music, and visual journaling were reported to be successful in facilitating collective metaphors, shared narratives, offering hope, and containing experiences of collective grief (Ma & Penner, 2018). A combination of therapeutic art making and psychodrama has also been known to facilitate group members' discussions of their experiences (Guzzino & Taxis, 1995). Such interventions can enhance peer support, emotional awareness, build resilience and reduce burnout often at very modest costs to organizations (Bell, Shanti, & Dalton, 2003, Ho et al., 2019, 2021; Potash et al., 2016).

Some aspects of the creative and expressive arts therapies can be adapted into accessible and scalable non-clinical psychosocial support initiatives. This can be done in an ethical ways that recognize the limits of non-clinical psychosocial support and knowing when to refer children and adults to professional mental health services. In particular, being responsive to local values and creative traditions can enable implementation of arts-based psychosocial interventions (Schininà et al., 2010). Creating this type of ethical non-clinical psychosocial support scalable public health intervention is thus the need and challenge that HEART has sought to meet over the past 14 years of innovation and practice.

Creating a Scalable Arts-Based Public Health Model of Psychosocial Support

Every community around the world has its own local arts practices that serve a range of purposes including strengthening social connections; storytelling and memory; noting milestones and festivals; and coping with adversity. For example, milestones like births of children, marriages, coming-of age, as well as deaths had associated rituals that integrated artistic activities. These expressive and creative practices and their therapeutic value were integrated into everyday life and members of the community had access to nonverbal forms of self-expression including visual arts, music, and dance. As such, the underlying value of these practices recognized the need to provide spaces for expression in times of joy but particularly in times of distress. As society industrialized and we moved away from our communities of origin, these creative practices that were part of everyday life slowly got removed from our lives. In the modern world, creative and expressive practices became the domain of professional artists, rather than each of us as humans.

Relatedly, in the twentieth century, the creative and expressive arts therapies also came to be established as professions. As creative practices became separate from our lives, their value for health and well-being came to exist instead as mental health professions. Given how distant everyday arts practices had become in our everyday lives, the creative and expressive arts practices became mental health professions to support the clinical needs of children and adults who were not able to benefit from traditional psychotherapies. In particular, the professions became an essential nonverbal therapeutic option in the mid-twentieth century. The mental health needs of special needs children in schools and of soldiers were not met by traditional psychotherapies or educational approaches. The principles behind these therapies were founded on several clinical antecedents such as the role of nonverbal expression as a pathway to psychosocial healing, which included creating a safe, nonjudgmental space for self-expression and engaging in our innate creative resources to problem solve. The idea was that when we are allowed to express our distress in verbal and nonverbal ways, we reduce isolation, shame, and guilt, and improve self-awareness.

To have tools for self-expression allows for self-regulation. HEART developed programming inspired by the creative and expressive arts therapies to offer ethical and high-quality psychosocial support to children and communities in need around the world. The model incorporates arts-based psychosocial support for emotional development, physical development of fine and gross motor skills, and cognitive development and group-based work to promote the development of social skills and of empathy with a focus on well-being and exercising agency and choice (self-esteem and self-confidence). The program allows for local adaptations that exercise creativity and imagination for experimentation, problem solving, and play primarily for children and youth, but also for the adults in their lives. The local context is respected, and integrating local values around creative self-expression is key to the work of HEART. Last and most importantly for sustainability, the model is customized to each location, recognizing and integrating local values for creative practices. As we mentioned previously, these creative and expressive aspects are natural ways that our predictive brain functions (for both children and adults). In addition, connecting individual expressive needs with local practices taps into our inherent creative instincts. Engaging in creative and expressive practices helps us naturally integrate movement, music, visual arts, drama, and storytelling into pathways for our emotional well-being, learning, and development.

Key Takeaways

Creative, expressive opportunities allow children and adults to experience safe ways to process, play, and navigate age-appropriate socioemotional and developmental milestones. Supporting adults and communities by tapping into local and regional resources of creative expression and strengths, recognizing vicarious traumas and compassion fatigue, and recognizing the resilience and opportunities for post-traumatic growth and transformation are impactful approaches to support children indirectly. Family caregivers and humanitarian workers can benefit from creative, expressive opportunities and ways to make meaning and reinforce social support and attachments, which in turn enables them to care adequately for their children.

Chapter 4

Healing and Education Through the Arts in Practice

Sara Hommel, May Aoun, Aida Bekic, and Dario Lipovac

The Creative Arts Therapies Influence on HEART

The Creative Arts Therapies refer to the combined fields of visual art therapy, music therapy, drama therapy, poetry therapy, and dance/movement therapy. Creative and expressive arts therapists are credentialed mental health providers who integrate the health promoting aspects of creative practices into psychotherapy practice. Other mental health practitioners can also use arts-based approaches in their clinical practices. Although different from the work of creative and expressive arts therapists, mental health professionals such as clinical psychologists, counselors, or clinical social workers often integrate arts-based approaches with other talk therapy approaches to enhance self-expression and communication within their psychotherapy and/or counseling practices. The professionalized study and practice of the creative arts therapies informed the design and implementation of HEART and helped to draw clear boundaries between nonclinical psychosocial support (such as HEART) and clinical mental health support (such as professional counseling or psychotherapy).

HEART uses many methods and techniques of the creative arts therapies to provide nonclinical psychosocial support to children and adults through creative group support processes. These techniques were especially identified to expand access to the psychosocial benefits of creative self-expression without misrepresenting or minimizing the very real and important clinical practices of psychotherapy for individuals with mental health needs. Most HEART facilitators are non-mental health professionals such as teachers or community facilitators. To create an expressive arts model that is simple and effective in nonclinical settings that adheres to the quality ethical standards of the creative arts therapies, it was necessary to **maintain specific approaches and techniques of the creative arts therapies, eliminate some, and adapt others.**

Ethical standards of the creative arts therapies that are **maintained** in HEART program facilitation reside primarily within a Do No Harm approach. This tactic includes a supportive approach to art making in which there is no right or wrong way to make art, individuals are in control of their own art-making process, and

DOI: 10.4324/9781003367529-5

no judgment of art creations takes place. It also includes an approach of inviting participation in both art making and visual and verbal sharing, meaning that participation is never forced. In addition, it includes supportive communication and the maintenance of confidentiality. The only time that confidentiality would not be upheld would be in a situation of concern over an individual's safety.

Ethical standards of the creative arts therapies that reflect the operational aspects of HEART also reflect the Do No Harm approach and focus on quality training protocols that ensure that facilitators are fully trained before they start the program, quality program standards that ensure regular and sustained support (frequency and duration of program sessions), and quality monitoring (or supervision) methods that ensure that facilitators are effectively supported and challenges are addressed appropriately throughout the programming cycle.

Creative arts therapy practices that are **not carried over** into HEART are those that would only be appropriate in a specialized mental health support setting. For example, an arts-assisted talk therapy approach that digs into individual experiences or attempts to uncover trauma and uses probing questions to respond to individual expressions (visual or verbal) would never take place in HEART. Facilitators are trained only to ask gentle generic questions to initiate sharing and discussion and never to dig into an individual's experience but rather to provide space for individuals to share as much as they like at their own pace. Also, there is no focus on identifying and working on a specific problem as there would be in a more traditional talk therapy approach. In HEART, the topics of the structured sessions are simple and generic. Although each individual person may relate to them in different ways based on personal experience, there is no focus on identifying or uncovering individual problems and then addressing those problems over time. Although HEART focuses on building basic stress-processing skills that will be beneficial to individual stress recovery, it is done in a generic way rather than focusing on specific issues or challenges of the individual. Notably, HEART does not use the word "therapy" in any of its trainings and programming. This distinction is important and essential to the ethical practice of arts-based psychosocial support in non-clinical settings.

Approaches of the creative arts therapies that are **adapted** for HEART include the training process, the exclusion of one-on-one support in favor of group support, and the role of referrals to specialized mental health services when needed. Professional art therapists go through years of training (both theoretical and practical) whereas HEART facilitators attend a 4.5-day introductory training followed by a period of supportive monitoring followed by a 2-day refresher training. HEART is always a group support model and is never used to provide individual support to one person, although facilitators may sometimes provide additional attention to an individual but always within the context of group facilitation. The outsourcing of specialized mental health support is not exclusive to HEART and is relevant for all MHPSS programming at

Save the Children. HEART facilitators are trained to understand potential signs of specialized mental health support needs and make referrals to specialized mental health service providers (outside of Save the Children). No diagnosis of mental health conditions ever takes place within the context of HEART, because the diagnosis and treatment of mental health disorders or the provision of more specialized mental health support such as professional counseling or psychiatric care is done through local specialized mental health services. Such services are usually provided through the local health-care system or by specialized medical International Nongovernmental Organizations (INGOs) in the local setting.

During the first few years of program development and piloting, a few key aspects of the program stood out as new concepts for many newly trained HEART facilitators who had no previous experience with expressive arts. To reinforce ethical programming approaches that seemed new or unusual to new facilitators, the program team developed a list of "HEART Guidelines" that are now provided to all HEART facilitators to remind them of key approaches discussed during their training. The list is not exhaustive but rather reflective of key ideas that seemed new for many participants and thus required reiteration throughout training and during the first stage of program piloting. After completing the introductory HEART training, all facilitators receive a HEART Facilitation Manual that includes the following list:

HEART GUIDELINES

1. Remember that "all art is good art" (do not judge or grade children's art). Do not teach children how to make art or correct the art they make. Allow them to explore the materials and art making on their own to be in control of their process.
2. Organize each activity ahead of time and have materials ready. Ensure enough time to finish all steps of the session and take care of the art materials and model this behavior for children – put materials away together after the session is finished.
3. Speak in a gentle tone of voice as it can help children to feel safe and supported.
4. Do not force children to participate. Invite them, encourage them, and thank them for their efforts, but do not force participation.
5. Do not assume what someone intends to communicate through their art. Invite participants to share and let them share as they want to (visually and/or verbally).
6. Be a good listener – give your full attention when someone shares.
7. Respect confidentiality.

8. No photos or videos without permission (and only at appropriate moments during preselected activities).
9. Prioritize your own self-care. Find your own way to process stress so that you are ready and able to support others.
10. Recognize that HEART facilitators are not therapists. They must refer to specialized mental health service providers if such support is needed.

HEART facilitators are also trained to use the local referral protocol.[1] This approach includes clarifying the logistics of the local referral mechanism and a basic orientation on how to identify signs that a child might require more specialized support than what is provided through HEART. Because the local referral system will vary from one location to another, it needs to be customized in each local programming context. Referrals can be related to mental health concerns, physical health or nutrition concerns, safety concerns, or other issues that should be addressed by a professional service provider outside of the HEART program.

In parallel to the focus on ensuring ethical standards through the work of HEART facilitators, there is also a process through which participants, including children, are engaged in ensuring the program's adherence to ethical programming standards. During the first phase of HEART in any new classroom or center, a "HEART Contract" is established between the facilitators and the participants. The HEART Contract is a set of agreements, designed collaboratively by the facilitators and participants, that lays out mutually agreed upon expectations of the program. This contract usually includes variations of the guidelines listed above, such as agreements on being good listeners, respecting confidentiality, recognizing that all art is good, and taking care of the materials. In some locations, the HEART Contract is a verbal agreement made during the first session and in other locations, it is written down and displayed on the wall as a reminder of key agreements to ensuring a good HEART process.

Launching HEART in a New Location

Before the HEART program can be integrated into a classroom or center, a process of consultation, planning, and coordination must take place to ensure that local conditions are conducive to quality programming standards. From the first step of planning to the final step of sustaining the program at the intended scale, the process of initiating HEART includes:

1. Consultation with local stakeholders
2. First introductory training (training of facilitators and program monitors/ supervisors)

3. First HEART pilot programming with monitoring
4. Review of monitoring feedback (and possible adjustments to local program)
5. First refresher training
6. Consultation with local stakeholders about HEART expansion (beyond the first pilot)
7. First training of trainers
8. Expansion of HEART beyond the first pilot (with monitoring)
9. Second refresher training and continued training of trainers process
10. Continued program expansion
11. Optional evaluation
12. Expansion, sustaining with quality, and scaling where appropriate.

Throughout the process of launching HEART in a new location, ethical programming standards are at the core of every step from initial consultations and planning to program training and resourcing to monitoring and evaluation.

Consultation

Consulting with local stakeholders focuses on determining whether local conditions are right for HEART. This process includes identifying appropriate settings such as schools or centers for HEART programming to take place and dedicated staff available to be trained as facilitators. It also includes confirming that there is appropriate time available in those settings to integrate HEART sessions into the weekly or bi-weekly schedule of the classrooms or centers. Attention is also paid to whether arts supplies are available to purchase at reasonable cost or whether local natural materials are available (at no or low cost) for making arts supplies[2] and how recycled materials can be used to supplement materials for arts activities. Discussions regarding the likelihood of the program becoming sustainable after the first phase of piloting is also discussed with particular focus on local financing and commitments of time and space for program facilitation. It is also during this initial consultation that confirmation of the local mental health referral system is discussed to ensure it is linked with the proposed HEART programming spaces.

Training

Once the consultation and planning processes are complete, the schools or centers have been selected for HEART program integration, and the facilitators are selected within the dedicated program spaces (often teachers, school counselors, or center facilitators), the first training is organized. Because most future HEART facilitators do not have previous experience with expressive arts or MHPSS, it is important to ensure that training is comprehensive. It is also important to ensure that all HEART facilitators receive training on the local mental health referral protocol before participating in HEART training.[3]

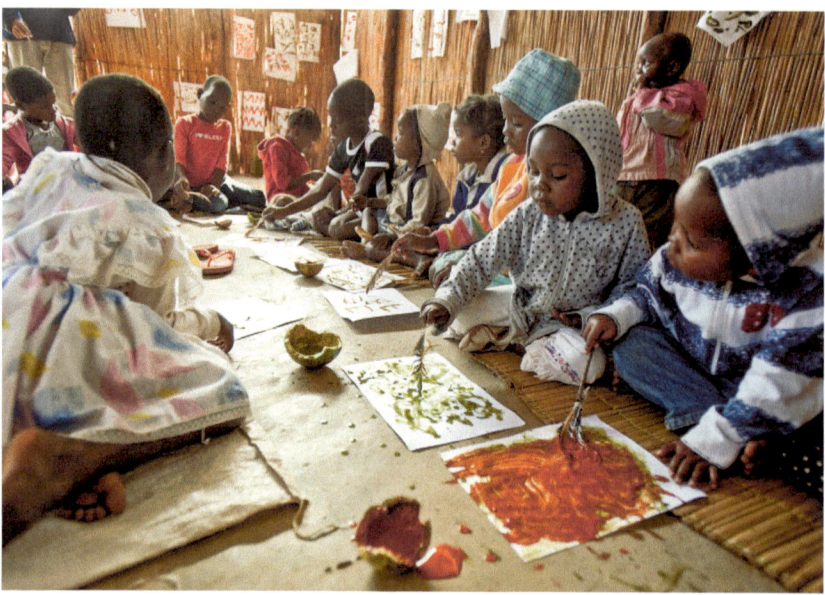

Figure 4.1 Children in Malawi paint with arts supplies made from local natural materials

Source: Save the Children

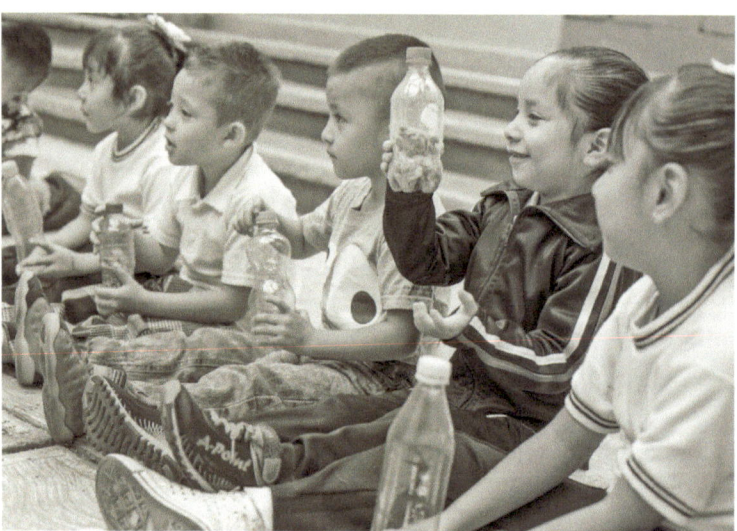

Figure 4.2 Children in Mexico prepare for a music activity using maracas made from recycled and natural materials

Source: Save the Children

To ensure that the HEART training process transfers a robust understanding of the importance of every aspect of the program, the training is intentionally designed to be significantly experiential. Over the course of 4.5 days, training participants are guided through a selection of full HEART sessions that use different arts modalities, focus on different topics, and have different logistical processes.[4] As such, participants experience the full process of different types of sessions. Each session includes relaxation activities, art making on a selected topic or theme, a sharing circle, grounding activities, and closing reflections. It is important for training participants to have time to experience full HEART sessions as many elements of the process are often new to those being trained. The training process includes time for questions and discussion on program components that may be new, confusing, or challenging for some participants.

> One of the primary challenges I encountered was persuading trainees (those we train to facilitate the program with children and adults) to embrace the concept of non-judgment and refrain from giving advice. In environments accustomed to training with firm positions on what's right or wrong, practicing supportive listening while grasping and implementing the principles of acceptance, non-judgment, and withholding advice proved to be difficult at the start. However, with consistent explanation, demonstration, support and follow-up, facilitators began to personally experience the transformative power of non-judgment and understand that child support programs are not always about lecturing and teaching, and facilitators and participants are equal companions in this process. Once you understand it, you understand the spirit of HEART – no judgement, only acceptance and support.
>
> (Global HEART Trainer)

Generally, the training is designed to alternate between short overviews and discussions of key program aspects and full HEART session experiences. In addition, after each HEART session is complete, the group discusses the session including ways it can be adapted to different age groups, different contexts, and different participant abilities.

To create a clear divide between the HEART sessions and the program discussions, the training room is carefully designed to have two separate spaces: one for HEART sessions and one for training overview and discussions on facilitation. This division allows participants to sit in the HEART session space and fully engage in the HEART session, without worrying about how they will facilitate the same process with children. Once the HEART session is finished, participants move to the discussion space to ask questions, discuss local considerations for session adaptation, and reflect on the future role they will play as facilitators.

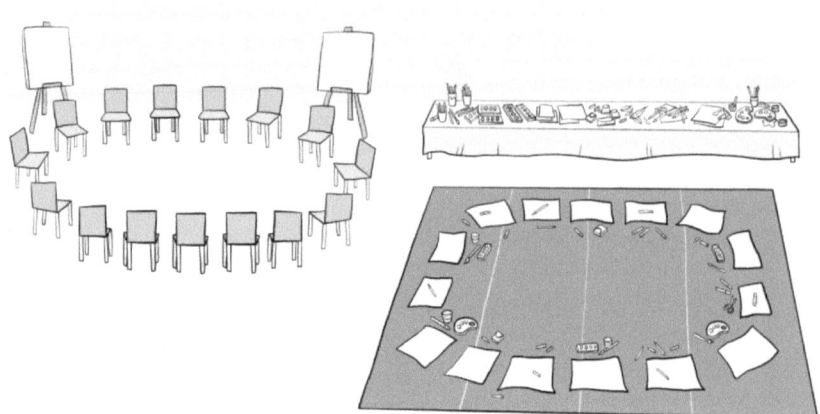

Figure 4.3 Training room illustration
Source: Kristyn S. Stickley

Throughout the course of the training, participants are exposed to diverse session content and process, logistical planning for session scheduling and organization, technical resource materials including a HEART Facilitator's Manual, and program monitoring tools. In addition to ensuring a quality training for future HEART facilitators, the experiential approach to the training also serves to directly deliver psychosocial support to the participants as they engage in each HEART session as themselves and experience the process as it relates to their own lives. The benefit of this experiential training process on individual staff well-being is discussed in more detail in Chapter 9.

HEART trainings typically include 20–30 participants and always have two trainers who co-facilitate the training process. One trainer leads each session while the other trainer assists, and they alternate roles throughout. The mandatory requirement that each training have two co-trainers ensures the psychosocial safety of the space and the psychosocial well-being of the trainers and participants because there are always two people to organize and set up the space (this is a significant amount of work), two people to co-manage a large group and divide when split into smaller groups, and two people to take turns leading challenging conversations. Because many of the conversations throughout the training can be emotionally "heavy," it is important that there are two trainers to share this work and support each other through the often rewarding yet exhausting training experience.

Global HEART trainers are often experienced global or regional[5] MHPSS staff members at Save the Children[6] who have gone through a Training of Trainers process that includes participating in one full cycle of HEART training (as a participant) followed by one or two cycles of co-facilitating HEART trainings with an experienced trainer who mentors and coaches the new trainer through the training process. Some HEART trainers who come from a non-MHPSS background such as education are provided additional MHPSS training, to complement their experience in HEART, and are always paired with an experienced MHPSS colleague to co-facilitate HEART trainings. The mix of MHPSS and education HEART trainers is especially useful when training teachers and school counselors, because the trainers themselves bridge the MHPSS and education pedagogical approaches that most directly link with each profession. Following the first 4.5-day introductory HEART training, a two-day refresher training is conducted approximately three to six months later. The intentional gap between the introductory training and refresher training allows the newly trained HEART facilitators several months of HEART programming experience before the refresher, so that the refresher training can address local challenges and celebrate local successes based on the interim period of HEART program piloting between the two trainings.

After the full cycle of HEART training (introductory training and refresher training) is complete, the first phase of program piloting has concluded, and the local HEART team has adjusted the local program adaptation as needed for local program standardization, a Training of Trainers process takes place in the local setting. Local trainers[7] are selected from the first cohort of local Save the Children staff, partner NGO staff, or facilitators that attended the full training cycle and were involved in the pilot either through HEART facilitation or monitoring of the HEART programming. They are selected based on demonstrated skills in HEART facilitation or monitoring as well as previous experience with training in complimentary program approaches (often MHPSS, education, or social work programming). The local Training of Trainers process is led by one of the global or regional HEART trainers who conducted the first training cycle and who is therefore familiar with the local program setting and local colleagues. The "master trainer" mentors and coaches the local trainers through training co-facilitation. This process is repeated as many times as the local trainers would like until they are comfortable continuing without the "master trainer" (often two rounds of coaching). Each Training of Trainers cycle (one introductory and one refresher training) includes 2–4 local trainers. The number of trainers trained in each cycle is small to ensure that the distribution of tasks throughout the training is substantial enough for each individual trainer to fully experience the entire process. This method ensures quality standards in HEART trainer training because the new trainers are involved in all aspects of the training while being closely coached by experienced trainers. This process also ensures that the expansion of the program is not delayed for trainer training because the Training of Trainer process happens during the training of new facilitators, so the expansion of local HEART trainers and local HEART facilitators happens simultaneously.

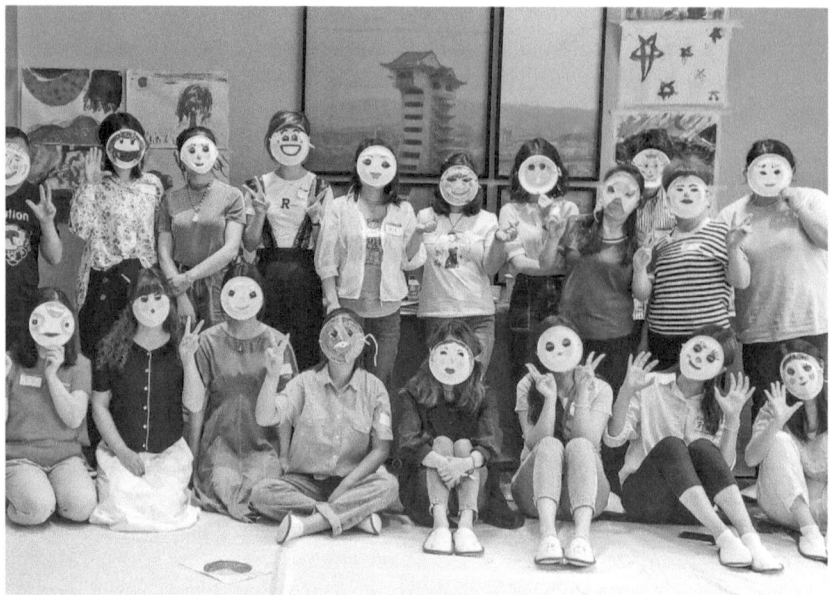

Figure 4.4 HEART training in China
Source: Save the Children

At the local level, the number of local trainers depends on the intended size and timeline of program expansion. Because every training requires two co-trainers, it is imperative to have multiple trainers available in the local setting to coordinate schedules for pairing trainers and to handle staff turnover over time. Most countries implementing HEART have between six and 30 local HEART trainers who are responsible for training hundreds or thousands of HEART facilitators. The process of initiating HEART in a new country with the support of global and regional trainers who eventually hand over the program to local trainers typically takes two years. The local and regional trainers are always available to support the country team again if needed, but with a large enough cohort of local trainers, the local team is often able to sustain and expand HEART without additional global or regional assistance.

Program Resources

A number of different programming resources exist to support the training of HEART facilitators, the facilitation of HEART with children, the facilitation of HEART with adults, the adaptation of HEART activities to support children with disabilities, the monitoring of HEART programming, and the evaluation of the impact of the HEART programming on different stakeholder groups. These include the following:

- Standard HEART Program Resources
  - Training Manual
  - Facilitation Manual
  - Monitoring Tools
  - Evaluation Tools
  - Guidance for Adapting to Support Children with Disabilities

- HEART Adaptation for Adults: Peer Support Groups
  - Training Manual
  - Facilitation Manual
  - Group Supervision Protocol
  - Monitoring and Evaluation Tools

To ensure quality ethical programming standards, HEART resources are not open source, meaning they are not available to use outside of the formal program process. The program resources are available only after training. HEART facilitators receive the program facilitation manual on the last day of the training program, during a discussion on local program adaptation, scheduling and sequencing HEART sessions, logistical planning, and program monitoring. Providing program resources only after local program planning and training are complete is part of the Do No Harm ethical approach. It ensures that the program is used only as intended by trained and supported facilitators within an appropriate programming context.

Program Piloting

Once the first cohort of HEART facilitators is trained, the first phase of program piloting starts. The first pilot is usually small, taking place within a few schools or centers. Facilitators receive ongoing support from the local Save the Children office including deliveries of arts supplies and advice on scheduling or adapting the programming space. As facilitators start implementing the program, usually one or two sessions per week, the local Save the Children technical staff, who are also trained to conduct HEART monitoring visits, check in with the facilitators to document challenges and successes. This supportive monitoring process serves to ensure continuous improvement of the program because challenges can be addressed quickly, and it also helps to document the local experience in ways that can support further adaptations to the local HEART programming model, which will be "standardized" after the pilot to ensure consistent programming during expansion.

One key process that takes place during the piloting period is the integration of local cultural art forms into the local program model. This step most often includes the use of local music and dance, particularly music and dance that is familiar and known to the children and that they find to be fun or relaxing. Music

and dance activities can be integrated into each session as relaxation or grounding activities or can be added to structured music or body movement activities
that exist within the standard program.

Another key process that takes place during the piloting period is the adaptation of activities to meet the local space. Although a process of adaptation
to local cultural norms[8] takes place before the pilot starts, the piloting period
often reveals a need for further adjustment to address logistical considerations
not previously identified. The way that HEART is organized in each classroom
or center varies based on the space and time available for HEART sessions. In
pre-school classrooms, the space is often easily arranged for different types of
activities, whereas in primary school classrooms, the space is often less flexible because desks and chairs need to be moved to clear open spaces. In classrooms with less flexible space adaptations, HEART facilitators often seek to use
alternative spaces within the school such as a gymnasium or empty classroom.
Different HEART activities require different logistical setups to facilitate individual, paired, or group art-making processes. Some of the most common session set-up formations are illustrated below.

After three to six months of piloting, a refresher training course is organized
for the same cohort of facilitators (only those who attended the introductory
training are invited to the refresher). The refresher training is intended to be
flexible in order to address local challenges and celebrate local successes from
the piloting period. The refresher training includes a session for feedback from
facilitators, which is added to the existing program monitoring data to support
the next phase of local program adaptation or expansion.

Once the local team is satisfied with the local HEART program model and
ready to expand beyond the first pilot, a new training of facilitators is organized
that includes a parallel Training of Trainers process as described above.

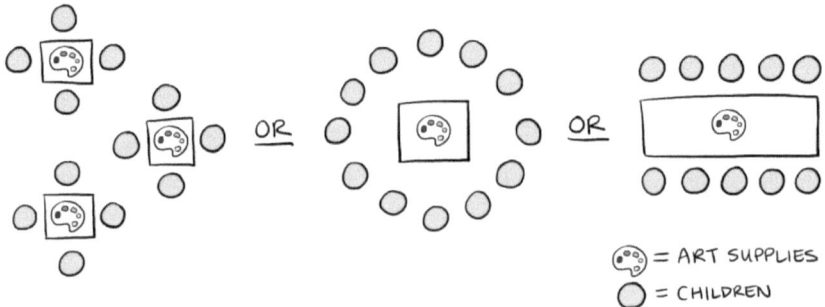

Figure 4.5 HEART classroom set-up options

Source: Kristyn S. Stickley

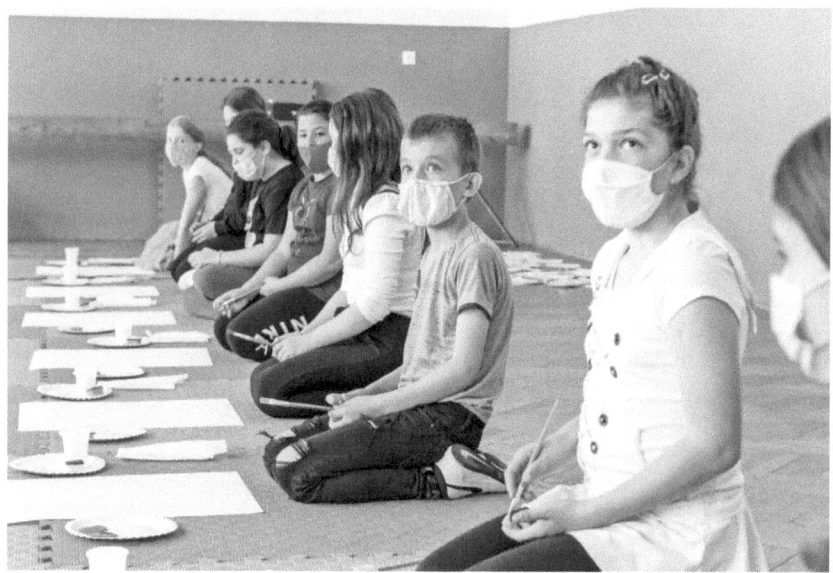

Figure 4.6 HEART in school gymnasium in Bosnia and Herzegovina

Source: Save the Children

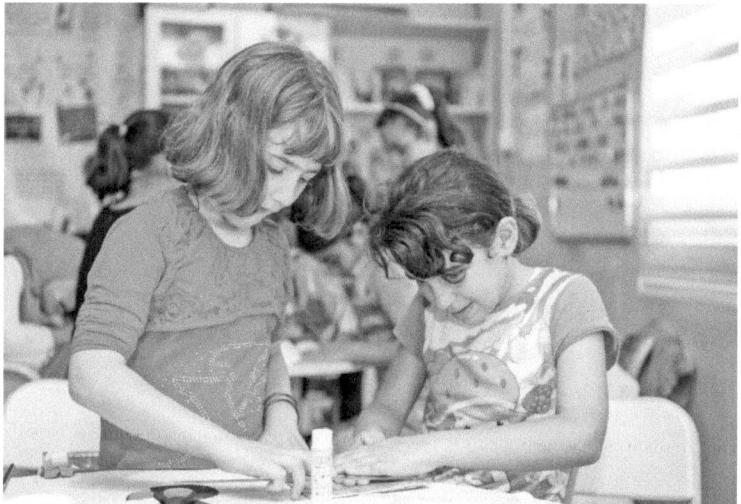

Figure 4.7 HEART in alternative learning classroom in Iraq

Source: Save the Children

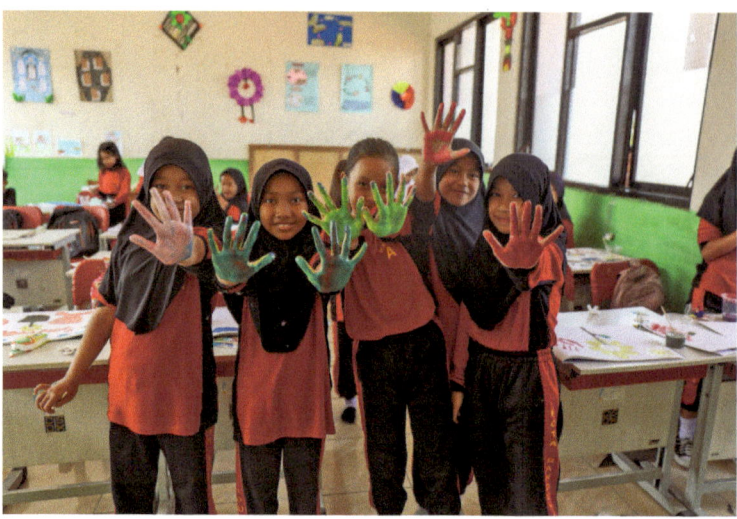

Figure 4.8 HEART in primary school classroom in Indonesia
Source: Save the Children

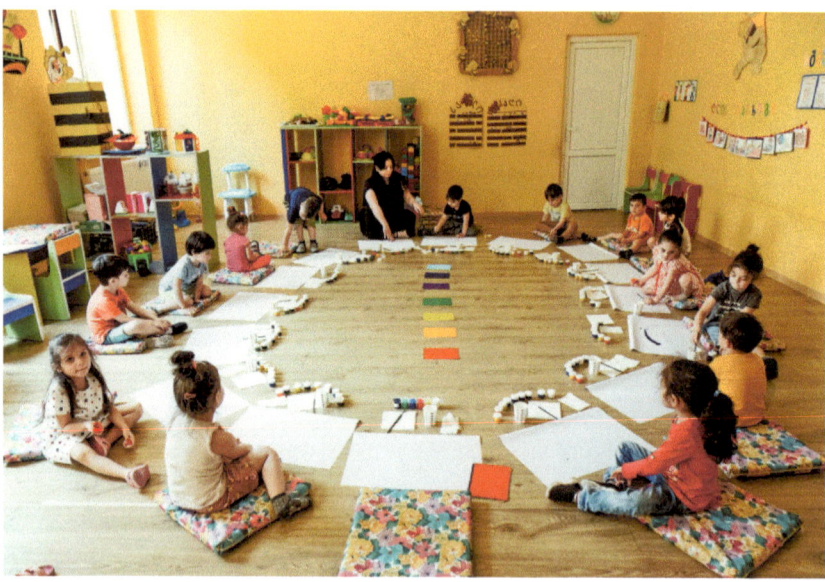

Figure 4.9 HEART in pre-school classroom in Georgia
Source: Save the Children

Monitoring

Regular technical program monitoring (bi-weekly or monthly) is conducted throughout the pilot period to collect feedback on challenges and successes to support continuous improvement and adaptation in the local context. The monitoring process continues after the piloting period is over but with less frequency (often monthly or quarterly). Two standard monitoring tools are provided. The first is a HEART Log, which is used by the HEART facilitator to document each HEART session they facilitate (with a special section to note any challenges or interesting experiences). The second is a Monitoring Visit Form for the HEART monitor to use during a visit to a specific class-room or center. The Monitoring Visit Form includes a checklist of logistical things to check on (such as the space used for HEART sessions and the quantity and quality of art supplies available) and an interview protocol to use to facilitate a supportive conversation with the HEART facilitator to document important aspects of their experience to date (with particular focus on challenges, successes, and additional support needs).

Post Pilot Expansion

Once the piloting period is complete, the refresher training is finished, the review of local monitoring data is conducted, and additional adjustments are made to the local program model, the local HEART team is then ready to expand beyond the pilot. Expansion requires new consultations and planning to identify additional schools and centers, organize new trainings of facilitators, procure and deliver arts supplies to new programming locations, and in some cases, for-malize agreements with local stakeholders including government ministries or local associations. After one or two rounds of Training of Trainers in parallel to training new cohorts of facilitators, the local HEART team is usually ready to continue program expansion without the support of global or regional HEART/MHPSS teams. Depending on partnerships between local stakeholder groups, the cost of HEART expansion is either funded by Save the Children or local government agencies or a mix of the two. More information about the financing of scaling HEART is discussed in Chapter 10.

Evaluation

Evaluation of HEART programming is optional[9] and is done only after the pilot period is complete and new expansion is underway. The quality ethical stand-ards that influence the program itself also influence the way the program is eval-uated. In HEART, there is no judgment, no right or wrong way to make art, and participation is voluntary. During the pilot period, facilitators find their way step by step, trying new activities they have never used before in their classroom or center. They document challenges and successes and receive support from Save the Children to adjust the program to fit the local context in the best way possible. It is important that the piloting process be supportive and flexible, without the added stress of formal evaluation. Thus, formal evaluation only takes place once the pilot is complete and the local HEART model has been reviewed and "standardized" for local expansion. Once expansion begins, formal evaluation can be considered where appropriate.

During the first 10 years of the HEART program, multiple evaluations were conducted using different types of evaluation tools and processes. Some tools produced useful data and some tools did not. Some tools were culturally appropriate and adjustable to the local context, and some were not. Some tools captured information relevant to the HEART program, and some did not. Some tools were expensive to use and some were not. As a result, a standardized HEART evaluation package was designed to include the most appropriate and effective evaluation tools. These tools include a Focus Group Protocol, a Key Informant Interview Protocol, and a Satisfaction Survey. All three tools are easily adjustable and culturally appropriate and capture information relevant to understanding the impact of HEART on different stakeholders[10] in different settings.

Ethical considerations that shaped the process of the HEART evaluation package design include the Do No Harm approach. To ensure that no one who participates in HEART feels judged through a formal evaluation, the evaluation process does not include the observation of HEART activities or any direct assessment of child well-being or possible secondary outcomes. This method includes the exclusion of pre- and post-testing methods that aim to capture change over time. Instead, the HEART evaluation package relies on observational data from adults who report on observed changes in children and on their professional or personal experience and subjective well-being as it relates to their participation in the program. These data are collected qualitatively and quantitatively, allowing for a process of triangulation that validates data from multiple tools across multiple locations.

All three HEART evaluation tools are used at the end of a program cycle, typically after six to nine months of programming with children or after two to four months of programming with adults. The Focus Group Discussions typically involve four to eight adult participants, one facilitator, and one note taker. The facilitator uses a list of basic open-ended questions to initiate group dialogue related to the observed impact on children, personal experience with the program, and a final question to invite any other information anyone would like to share. Key Informant Interviews use questions similar to those used in the Focus Groups but are conducted one on one. The Satisfaction Survey is most often used with adult HEART programming including both the Parent and Caregiver Peer Support Groups and Staff Peer Support Groups and can be used either as a monitoring tool or as an evaluation tool. It contains several specific questions related to the logistics and facilitation of the local program, which are used for quality program monitoring. It also contains several questions related to personal subjective well-being and social connectedness (indicators of psychosocial well-being), which are used to demonstrate program impact. Results of HEART evaluation in different countries is discussed in more detail in later chapters.

HEART Programming Variations

HEART is primarily used to support children and youth ages 4–18 and is designed to enhance their psychosocial well-being, development, and learning. HEART sessions focus on relaxation, stress processing, understanding emotions, emotional regulation, confidence building, problem solving, conceptualizing the future, and supportive group communication. HEART takes place through weekly sessions over an extended period, often six to nine months, following the school year or other organized child-support setting.

The adaptation of HEART to support adults, including parents and caregivers, takes place through weekly or bi-weekly sessions for 2–6+ months (scheduling and duration are customized in each local setting). Parents and caregivers of children attending school or community-based programs supported by Save the Children are invited to join groups of 10–15 adult peers. Through the support group sessions, with the guidance of trained facilitators, they explore themes related to stress processing, supportive communication, normalization of feelings and emotions, future orientation, and self-care practices. They also explore methods for supporting the psychosocial well-being of children so that they can better support children at home (more information on the Parent and Caregivers Peer Support Groups adaptation of HEART is in Chapter 8). A similar version of the program is used to support adult staff including teachers, health workers, social workers, and Save the Children staff members (more information on the Staff Peer Support Groups adaptation of HEART is in Chapter 9).

In some programming locations or contexts, additional variations of the HEART program are sometimes necessary. This approach includes starting with a Condensed HEART Program[11] several months before initiating the full standard program with children. The condensed program is used only in settings in which the full program is not possible, either due to logistical restrictions or the need for reduced program content. Logistical restrictions could be related to the local security situation or social distancing protocols. The need for reduced program content could either be related to limited access to arts materials (or natural resources to make arts supplies) or to the need for gentle and recreational focused arts activities due to a high stress context in which the full program could be overwhelming for some participants and facilitators. Examples of the use of the Condensed HEART Program include community center-facilitated programming during the COVID-19 pandemic that required reduced center hours and physical distancing between children within the center, and school-, center-, or shelter-facilitated programming during armed conflict in Ukraine and Syria. The Condensed Program is always used temporarily, and once conditions allow, it transitions to the full program.

Another variation that is used either during logistical restrictions or as a supplement to the full program, is HEART at Home. HEART at Home is described in a short pamphlet that includes a few examples of simple expressive arts activities that families can do together at home. The HEART at Home pamphlet along with a bag of arts supplies is sometimes distributed to parents who attend the Parent and Caregiver Peer Support Groups or to children who participate in HEART at a center or school; it can also be distributed directly to homes or shelters during mandatory lockdowns such as those experienced during armed conflict or an infectious disease outbreak.

Additional examples of HEART programming variations and more specific details related to the use of HEART for different age groups, children with disabilities, parents and caregivers, and staff are explored in more detail in Chapters 5–9.

Sustaining and Scaling Up

The experience of sustaining and expanding HEART programs varies across countries and contexts. In some locations, HEART is intended to integrate fully into a local school system and sustain indefinitely. In other locations, HEART is intended to be a temporary program, for example, one that is used in a community center for six months during an emergency response. In many locations, multiple variations of HEART are used simultaneously to meet the needs of different populations at different times; in other contexts, only one version of the program takes place. Specific examples of sustaining and scaling up HEART in different countries are discussed in more detail in Chapter 10.

Key Takeaways

The goal of HEART is to improve the psychosocial well-being of children, parents, caregivers, teachers, and other child-support workers. The dual approach of supporting children and their caregivers within the community (both at home and at school) is explored in more detail in the next part of this book. Chapters 5 –9 explore the experience of HEART in supporting children of different ages, children with special needs, parents and caregivers, and staff in different contexts and settings around the world. Chapter 10 explores the scaling up of HEART in specific countries and Chapter 11 explores lessons learned and future plans for Healing and Education through the Arts across the globe.

Notes

1 The local referral system often includes coordination between education, health, social, and protection systems in the local setting. Each location will have a logistical pathway through which an individual in need of specialized support is linked with the appropriate service to provide that support. For HEART, this means that facilitators are trained to know who the referral focal points are within their programming context (e.g., school, community center) and how to contact those focal points and ensure a safe and supportive process for referring a child for specialized support.

2 Making arts supplies from locally available natural materials often includes digging up and sterilizing natural clay for sculpting, making paint brushes out of sticks or sterilized feathers, and making paint by mixing crushed berries, leaves, or charcoal with water and natural powders.

3 Local mental health referral training often includes a combination of training approaches involving local Safe Identification and Referral protocols, Psychological First Aid, or similar approaches alongside logistical operating procedures.

4 Each training period includes at least one session that uses each art modality including drawing, painting, sculpture, music, drama, dance or body movement, book making, and a mixed-modality session. It also includes different logistical processes including individual art making, making art in pairs, and group work. It is important to note that sharing circles, after the art-making process is complete, is done as one group, with individuals, pairs, or groups invited to share their artwork, feelings, ideas, and experiences as they like.

5 Global staff members work across multiple countries and regions. Regional staff members work across multiple countries within one region.

6 MHPSS staff members at Save the Children typically have a professional background in social work, psychology, education psychology, or a related field.

7 Local HEART trainers are either local Save the Children national staff members who work within their country or local staff members from a partner organization such as a local NGO, government agency, or HEART program location such as a school or community center (schools are often managed by the Ministry of Education and community centers are often managed by a local NGOs).

8 Adaptations of the program based on local cultural norms often include logistical considerations for same-gender groups, the designation of specific animals or symbols to be included or excluded in specific activities, and in some cases, the removal of music and dance (for example, in religiously conservative communities where music and dance are forbidden).

9 Evaluation (formal research) of HEART is optional in local program settings. This means that Save the Children does not require the program to be evaluated in every individual programming location or country. HEART has been formally evaluated multiple times and will continue to be evaluated in different ways in different settings, but it is not mandatory for each HEART setting to run formal evaluations. Monitoring is mandatory to ensure quality programming standards, but formal evaluation is not compulsory.

10 HEART evaluation tools aim to capture information that demonstrates an impact on children, parents, and other caregivers and on staff including HEART facilitators.

11 The Condensed HEART Program contains approximately 20% of the full program. The activities included are mostly simple dramatic play relaxation activities, free arts activities using basic arts supplies such as paper and drawing utensils, and a few simple structured activities with generic topics that are positive and joyful.

Chapter 5

HEART in Early Childhood

Amy Parker, Carolyn Alesbury, Phoebe Marabi,
Ana Lagidze, and Laila Sabbagh

Early Childhood Development

Early childhood, which extends through age 8, represents a period of significant social and physical development for children as they learn to navigate the world around them. During this period, children become increasingly aware of and able to distinguish between themselves and others, setting the stage for the attachments they will form throughout their lives. Their lived experiences as they interact with their families, caregivers, and wider environments throughout this period of development have been shown to influence children's cognitive, social, emotional, and physical outcomes well into their futures (Barnett, 1985; Zeanah et al., 2017).

Brain development begins two weeks after conception and, along with genetics, is impacted by environmental factors, such as nutrition and maternal health (Tierney & Nelson, 2009). Although the brain does not complete its development until young adulthood, the foundations for memory, decision making, and emotional skills are laid primarily in the early years, and early experiences have been proven to heavily influence developmental outcomes (Tierney & Nelson, 2009; Zeanah et al., 2017). Stressors that children live through during this sensitive period can, so long as they are minor, help build their resiliency and coping strategies (Shonkoff, 2010). However, for some children, stress reaches toxic levels as they live through extended and intense adverse experiences, such as conflict, abuse, and famine, along with a lack of mitigating support and stability. For these children, the impact of such adverse experiences on the development of their brain can result in damaging lifelong repercussions on learning, behavior, and physical and mental health (Shonkoff & Garner, 2011; Franke, 2014). Research has shown that adverse experiences and toxic stress can lead to underdeveloped neural connections, particularly in the areas of the brain responsible for executive function skills (Tierney & Nelson, 2009). At the same time, the area of the brain that controls the child's ability to respond to fearful stimuli overdevelops neural connections, which can lead to heightened responses to future stressors (Tierney & Nelson, 2009). In order to cope, the

DOI: 10.4324/9781003367529-6

brain may disengage during adverse experiences as physical, mental, and emotional energy is used to keep difficult emotions at bay, which may lead to emotional detachment and disassociation (Hussain, 2010). Young children may also experience difficulty expressing their emotions, because memories of adversity and trauma are stored in the nonverbal regions of the limbic system, and they may not yet have the language skills to fully communicate what they are feeling (Hussain, 2010).

Children's early experiences can also impact their physical development and well-being. As they progress through gross motor and fine motor skill development, young children gain greater levels of control over their bodies, although this process can be delayed or disrupted for children with some types of chronic health conditions and/or disabilities. Physical developments are also influenced by biological responses to stress and by environmental factors including exposure to toxins and household crowding (Shonkoff & Garner, 2011; Franke, 2010; Ferguson et al., 2013). Additionally, adverse experiences and toxic stress during the early childhood years have also been found to impact health in later life, including dramatically increased odds of physical health problems as adults (Shonkoff & Garner, 2011).

Equally important to children's development are the positive experiences and protective factors that help mitigate some of the stressors in their young lives. Protective factors can come from many sources in a child's life. Under Bronfenbrenner's ecological systems theory, children are impacted by nested systems of influence, ranging from those closest to them (such as their family and caregivers), to those that exist at a higher level (such as the policy environment). Within this theory, preschool teachers and classmates would fall under the microsystem—the system closest to the child—at the same level as the child's family (Bronfenbrenner, 1979). Protective factors at the macro level may include protective social policies, while at the micro level they may include supportive relationships, unconditional love, presence of trusted adults, social engagement, opportunities to learn, and rewarding activities. It is at this level that the HEART program aims to support young children.

HEART in Early Childhood Settings

HEART as a Protective Approach for Psychosocial Well-Being in Young Children

HEART is a nonclinical intervention that provides psychosocial support for children; at the early childhood level, this support takes place primarily through center-based activities for students aged 3 and older. The design of the HEART approach is intentionally structured and predictable to build a supportive environment and to provide opportunities to regularly engage in creative activities with others, establishing a network of trusted peers and adults. Providing regular and predictable supportive experiences for children over time is an example of Protective and Compensatory Experiences (PACES), providing protective experiences involving productive activities and supportive relationships with adult caregivers and peers (Hays-Grudo & Morris, 2020). There is a growing body of evidence that suggests that play, including expressive arts, can help support children to develop the skills they need to cope with stress and adversity, including being able to make sense of uncertainties (Yogman et al., 2018). Particularly for children from economically disadvantaged contexts, the arts can also lead to positive impacts in terms of stress reduction, emotional regulation, verbal communication, impulse control, self-esteem, and socioemotional readiness to learn (Brown et al., 2017; Brown & Sax, 2013; Klorer & Robb, 2012).

HEART's use of the expressive arts is especially powerful for younger children who may not be able to verbalize how they are feeling and therefore for whom traditional, talk-based therapeutic support is less effective (Levick, 1983; Rubin, 2010). With the focus on the process rather than on the end result, and the mantra that "all art is good art," young children build confidence in a space where they will not be judged as inadequate or wrong. Ultimately, HEART activities are designed to provide three main therapeutic benefits known to be associated with art: (a) the physical nature of making art is a form of relaxation and thus helps to mitigate anxiety; (b) the process of creating art is a personal and introspective event; and (c) by discussing the process and the art afterward along with the specific topic or theme of the activity, children are able to reflect on their art-making process, ideas, experiences, feelings, and emotions.

In addition to the benefits outlined above, HEART also promotes a sense of personal agency for young children. By allowing children to choose how they participate in activities and what they create, the program maximizes individual decision making and uses culturally, socially, and age-appropriate resources, examples, and activities to establish a supportive and nonjudgmental environment. Whereas facilitators are trained to respond appropriately to children demonstrating or disclosing upsetting experiences, there is also a focus on children being children and having fun. This combination of safe, engaging, and empowering activities facilitated by trained adults and carried out in safe and supportive environments, works to ensure that even the youngest children have the time and space to regain a little bit of control in what are often highly chaotic situations. They are given time to breathe—and to learn how to process and communicate stress and explore ways to self-regulate.

HEART in Practice in Preschool Classrooms

The most common setting for HEART in early childhood is the preschool classroom. Given that preschool education is significantly less formalized than primary or secondary education globally, there is often significant flexibility within a preschool classroom that is usually not present in primary or secondary school

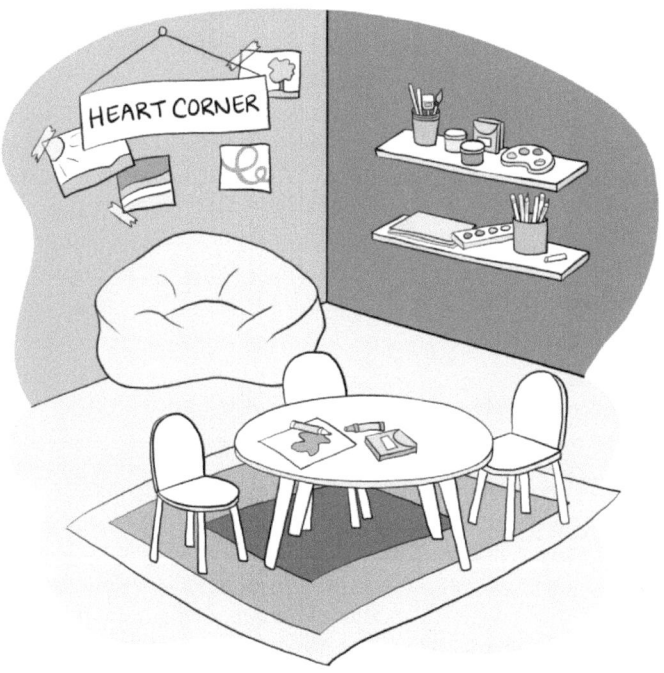

Figure 5.1 HEART corner
Source: Kristyn S. Stickley

settings. As a result, integrating HEART into preschool classrooms often faces significantly fewer logistical challenges than formal school settings for older children, meaning that HEART sessions can usually be scheduled at least twice per week (and often more than twice per week) in the preschool classroom.

In addition to scheduling flexibility, preschool classrooms are also more likely to experience flexible space configuration because they are not dependent on the typical desk and chair setup of a formal primary or secondary school setting. As a result, preschool classrooms are more likely to have comfortable open floor seating for group arts activities or tables that can fit multiple children for group activities. The physical setup of a HEART integrated preschool classroom is also more likely to benefit from a "HEART Corner," a dedicated, permanent space with arts materials and comfortable seating for up to a few children at a time, for self-guided use by children when they feel overwhelmed and in need of extra time and space, alone or with the support of their teacher, for creative self-expression.

Despite significant gains in the global expansion of preschool programming in recent decades, universal preschool education is still significantly underprioritized. The latest pre-COVID-19 pandemic data indicate that in low-income countries, only one in five children have access to preschool education (UNICEF, 2019) and for those who do have access, the quality of services available varies significantly from one location to another, dependent on a variety of factors including infrastructure, sustainable funding, materials, and teacher training. In many locations where Save the Children works, preschool teacher professionalization is a significant challenge. As a result, Save the Children partners with governments, NGOs, community associations, and other strategic stakeholders to provide additional training for preschool teachers and supplies for preschool classrooms, in both formal and informal preschool education settings. The following examples demonstrate the role of HEART in preschool education in four countries.

HEART in Action in Humanitarian Response: Examples from Tanzania and Nigeria

The use of HEART in long-term emergency response programming, such as in internally displaced people (IDP) and refugee camps, includes the integration of the program into preschools and community centers that support children under the age of 8. The logistics of child support programming in long-term emergency response varies from one location to another. Often, there is overlap between programming for early childhood (under 8 years old) and childhood (under 18 years old) as the 6- to 8-year-old age group can logistically fall into both early childhood and childhood programming spaces. In many IDP or refugee camp settings, Save the Children supports preschools and community centers (often referred to as Child Friendly Spaces or CFS) where HEART is integrated. In some locations, children aged 6 and under attend the preschool, and children aged 6 and over attend the CFS. In other locations where preschools either do not exist or do not have room to accommodate all children in the designated age range, the CFS is set up to have programming for early childhood age groups in addition to the older age range. In contexts where CFS supports both age groups, it is possible that in some locations CFS facilitators are dedicated to specific age groups and in other locations they work with both age ranges. As a result, training of HEART facilitators can be done in ways that cover the entire age range or can be customized to specific age groups when appropriate.

Two examples of the integration of HEART into long-term humanitarian response settings that include early childhood support programming are in CFS in IDP settings in northeast Nigeria and in preschools in refugee camps in western Tanzania. In Nigeria, the HEART sessions are implemented for different age groups at different times in the CFS by the same facilitators (facilitators trained to adapt activities to different age groups). In Tanzania, HEART is integrated into preschools for the early childhood group and into CFS for the older group, and each setting has its own facilitators who are trained together. It is important to note that in both countries, facilitators in both the preschools and CFS are members of the local community, meaning that just like the children, they are refugees or IDPs who also live in the camp and whose lives are also in transition.

For families who are internally displaced due to armed violence in northeast Nigeria, CFS in the IDP camps include HEART scheduled for different age groups at different times. For Congolese and Burundian families living in refugee camps in western Tanzania, preschools implement HEART for the early childhood age group. In both countries, HEART is very popular with children and facilitators. HEART facilitators in both countries reported increased attendance. In both countries, facilitators also reported that children are extremely proud of the art they create and often take it home to share with their families, which led to parents and caregivers visiting the preschools and CFS to share how excited their children are to bring home their art creations.

HEART facilitators in both countries also reported observing increased confidence and increased empathy in children. These two points of feedback seem to be linked because children were seen to be becoming increasingly patient and empathetic with each other during sharing circles. Over time, children were noted to have increased confidence in participating in the sharing circle. As the sessions progressed, many more children became more comfortable sharing, especially those who seemed shy and withdrawn during earlier sessions. Some parents and caregivers, especially in Nigeria, reported that their children became more expressive and communicative at home after participating in HEART for several months.

Because humanitarian contexts are often unstable or in constant transition, there are significant challenges to sustaining quality HEART programming. In unstable security environments, such as northeast Nigeria, there are sometimes travel restrictions that prevent local Save the Children staff members from traveling to the CFS locations to deliver arts materials or conduct program monitoring visits. In settings that are in constant transition, such as refugee camps in western Tanzania, trained HEART facilitators often leave once they can return to their home country, so staff turnover is significant and requires repeated training of new facilitators to sustain HEART in the preschools and CFS. Given the unstable environments in humanitarian settings, there is significantly less opportunity, than in development settings, for standardizing a local HEART model as the program is constantly adapting to new challenges and context transitions. This unstable programming setting also limits opportunities for evaluating the local program and sustaining a stable program model over time. Despite the many challenges, arts-based psychosocial support in such vulnerable settings is extremely important and impactful and remains a core focus of HEART around the world. Providing children in such vulnerable settings with quality PACES can have positive lifelong impacts on their development, learning, and well-being.

HEART in Action in Development Contexts: Mexico and Georgia

Mexico

Setting the Scene. The stressors impacting young children in Mexico are numerous and complex. Many families are faced with significant economic challenges because, despite falling levels in recent years, over one-third of the population still lives in a state of multidimensional poverty (World Bank, 2023). Many children are also exposed to violence at a young age because Mexico currently experiences the second highest magnitude of homicide in the region, second only to Brazil (UNODC, 2023). It is in this context that the HEART program aims to strengthen the protective factors that support children in their early years of development in Mexico.

HEART was initially launched in preschools in Mexico City in 2015, providing expressive arts programming to children who were regularly exposed to domestic and community violence and to household poverty. To date, the program has been active in 136 preschools, reaching 120 adult facilitators and

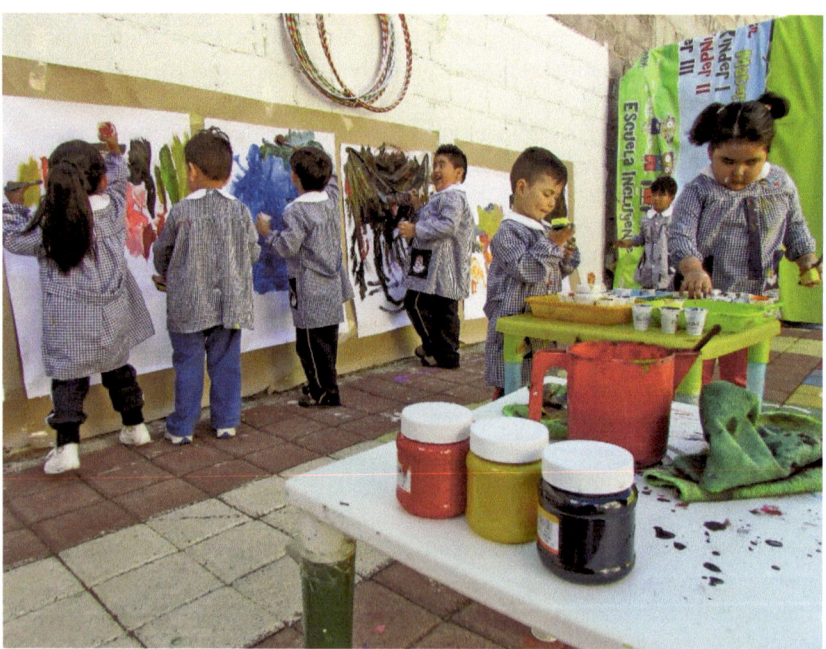

Figure 5.2 Children painting during a HEART session at their preschool in Mexico

Source: Save the Children

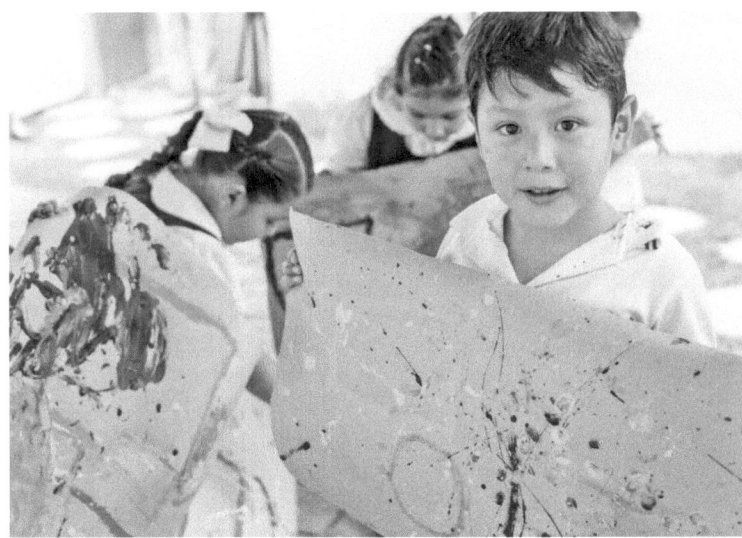

Figure 5.3 Children participate in HEART at their preschool in Mexico
Source: Save the Children

over 10,000 children. The community-based preschools where HEART is operating were originally established by local mothers to provide safe spaces where young children could play, learn, and receive emotional support from reliable and caring adults. Following the HEART training and distribution of materials, preschool teachers began leading children through weekly HEART activities and established "HEART Corners" in each classroom, where students could find comfortable seating and art supplies. Children are encouraged to use the space at any time during the day if they are feeling stressed or inspired, and teachers make themselves available if the children wish to share their art or talk about their feelings. By adding HEART Corners in addition to the weekly HEART activities, the preschool teachers maximize children's sense of agency over their participation in the program and help children gain a sense of control in light of potentially stressful home and community circumstances.

What Has HEART Meant for Children? The safe space established by HEART and the opportunity for children to express themselves through art together with trusted peers and adults have led to positive changes among the young children targeted by the program. A 2019 evaluation found that both parents and teachers noticed that children's emotional regulation and expression had improved over several months of participation in the program (Pisani et al., 2021). The children demonstrated an increased ability to calm down and follow instructions and exhibited improvement in social connections with other children (Pisani et al., 2021).

For individual children participating in the program, HEART has led to noticeable changes in their behavior and well-being. Mateo,[1] a young boy who lives primarily with his grandparents while his parents work, was initially a withdrawn child at preschool. In addition to the uncertainty of not seeing his parents for up to a week at a time, he had also witnessed their acrimonious divorce and associated fighting in the home. At preschool, his teachers noticed Mateo becoming withdrawn and demonstrating signs of anxiety, which manifested through biting his nails, getting angry or aggressive with his peers, and isolating himself from other children. Mateo had even stopped participating in organized classroom activities by the time HEART began in his preschool. Following his gradual exposure to HEART, however, teachers began to notice some small changes; Matteo became slightly more vocal, more willing to participate, and would briefly share his artwork after an activity. Over time, he became more engaged in the classroom and eventually stopped biting his nails, smiled more, and began to participate in not only HEART activities but also in other types of play and games with his classmates.

Similarly, Sofia,[2] a young girl coping with the unexpected death of her grandfather, had become withdrawn and fearful at preschool. Her teachers recognized that Sofia needed to process her experience and encouraged her to spend as much time as she wanted in the HEART Corner (whenever she felt sad or overwhelmed during the day). The walls of the HEART Corner in her preschool are colorfully painted with the sun, clouds, and trees, and comfortable seats and art supplies are available for the children to use. Sofia would spend approximately 15 minutes each day in the HEART Corner, drawing pictures of her grandfather, writing him letters, and telling him how much she loved and missed him. Through this physically and psychologically safe environment, Sofia began to open up more with her peers and teachers, even more so than she had at home. Over time, Sofia found that she needed to go to the HEART Corner less frequently and was able to re-engage more in class. One day, Sofia drew a picture for her grandfather, and when she held it to her chest, she left an imprint of a heart over her own heart on her skin and clothing. Her teachers heard her say: "I feel that my grandfather is already on my heart. I don't need this paper anymore because I have it on me. And whenever I want to talk to my grandfather, I know I have him in my heart." Her teachers could see the progress Sofia was making through her grief and felt that HEART helped her to cope with her loss.

What Has HEART Meant for Parents and Other Adult Caregivers? Parents and caregivers are exposed to the same stressors faced by their children, in addition to the stress of caring for their families. To help address these challenges, the Mexico City preschool teachers who were trained in HEART began to facilitate sessions directly with their students' parents and caregivers. Through peer support groups, the teachers worked with parents to provide them with sessions that delivered direct psychosocial support that focused on their well-being and with sessions focused on how best to support their children during times of stress. This approach helped strengthen relationships between parents and teachers at the preschool and within the broader community. Interviews and focus group discussions with parents in Mexico City conducted at the 2019 evaluation found that after HEART, parents reported feeling closer to their children and being better able to respond to their children's needs. Parents also reported that HEART activities had helped them to manage their own stress and had improved their own emotional expression (Kaimal et al., 2022).

What Has HEART Meant for Teachers? As mentioned previously, the Mexico City preschools participating in the HEART program were initially established by the mothers of children in the community. Over the past decade, the parent–preschool teachers have been steadily professionalizing themselves through participating in numerous trainings provided by Save the Children and other organizations in Mexico. These efforts have led to increased quality of services provided to children and to increased personal growth among the teachers themselves. From HEART trainings in particular, teachers have expressed an improvement in their own well-being as well as an increased ability to express themselves, process emotions, and manage stress (Pisani et al., 2021). In the 2019 evaluation, teachers also indicated that the program helped them relate better to children and equipped them to help children process stress in creative rather than destructive ways (Kamal et al., 2022). Some teachers even reported that they had begun teaching HEART techniques to their families to improve relationships at home (Pisani et al., 2021). One teacher, Victoria, summed up her learning from HEART as "be the adult you needed when you were a child." She felt that the HEART program has helped her better accompany children as they express themselves and their emotions. After her first four years with the program, Victoria reported that she allowed her inner child to have fun while creating a safe and trusting environment for children. "This fills me with immense pride, and joy and keeps me committed to continue creating and promoting a caring classroom to reach more and more spaces where empathy and love can continue to support children to flourish."

Georgia

Setting the Scene. Although violence levels are lower than those in Mexico, many young children in Georgia are exposed to economic stressors, with over 17% of the population living below the national poverty line (World Bank, 2023b). Additionally, children with disabilities living in Georgia are often unable to obtain the necessary social services, and many remain largely "invisible" in the broader community (UNICEF, 2017a). Access to quality preschool services

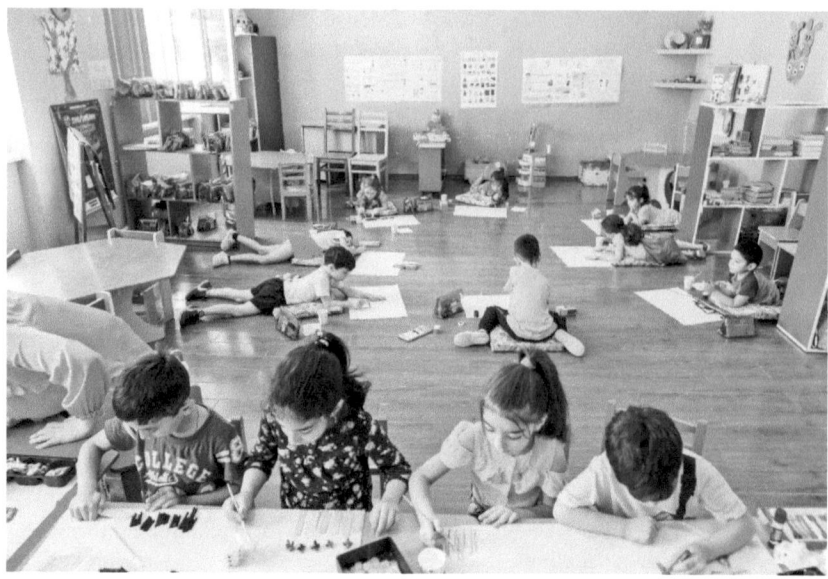

Figure 5.4 Children participate in HEART at their preschool in Georgia

Source: Save the Children

is also a challenge. Even though the government has mandated universal free preprimary education, nearly half of the eligible children are still not attending early childhood development programs (UNICEF, 2017b). Enrollment rates are even lower for children with disabilities, those from ethnic minorities, and those living in rural areas (UNICEF, 2017b).

Children who are able to enroll in preschool are met with high student-to-teacher ratios, teachers who have received limited training, and a lack of educational and play resources. Further complicating the quality of preschool education in Georgia is the low professional status given to preschool teachers, which is reflected in their low salaries. Preschool centers therefore face difficulties recruiting and retaining highly qualified teachers, and many of the teachers who are present do not have access to professional development opportunities. At the same time, the education system has been decentralizing since 2005, when governance of preschools was transitioned from the national government to the municipal level. The adaptation of municipalities to their new responsibilities has been slow and complicated by new policy developments aimed at improving quality, access, and equity in preschool. It is within this evolving environment that HEART was first introduced in 2019.

Initially launched in Tbilisi and Rustavi municipal preschools, HEART's goal was to improve existing preschool services by training preschool teachers, providing arts materials to their classrooms, and ensuring that students had access to regular interactive expressive arts programming. The approach included a specific focus on children with disabilities, those with special education needs, and those with developmental delays. Most preschool teachers surveyed in the initial weeks after the first HEART training reported that they conducted relaxation activities and energizers with students daily, and used structured sessions and free arts sessions at least once per week. However, as they became more proficient with HEART and began to see the positive impact on their students, they gradually found opportunities to integrate structured sessions and free arts sessions more frequently, with some teachers reporting that they conducted structured and free arts sessions up to five times per week. As of December 2023, HEART has been implemented in 155 preschools in Tbilisi—which includes over half of all the preschools in the city—as well as in 22 preschools in Rustavi and 37 in Kutaisi. A total of 755 facilitators have been trained, and 30,000 children have participated in the program across all three locations. Building on the successes of the program, the government of Georgia has planned to scale up HEART and institutionalize it at a national level.

What Has HEART Meant for Children? A 2021 evaluation of HEART in Georgia used interviews, focus groups, and online surveys with 75 preschool teachers to better understand the impact of the program on the lives of those it reached. According to the teachers, children made visible progress in the development of their social-emotional skills, cognitive skills, speech and language capabilities, communication skills, independence, and adaptability (Save the Children, 2021a). HEART activities provided students with an opportunity to share their emotions and practice working in groups together with others. Ultimately the teachers reported that students were able to better manage their stress, were more engaged in the learning environment overall, and became more active and courageous (Save the Children, 2021a). Children were also more open about sharing their opinions with peers and adults, and teachers noted that students were very respectful of one another—not discussing what others had shared during HEART as they might have done during other activities (Save the Children, 2021a). Teachers also reported that students talked about HEART so often with their parents that parental engagement in their preschool education seemed to increase as a result.

For children with disabilities, HEART activities were a particularly enriching experience, helping them to develop skills alongside their peers. For example, one teacher highlighted the case of a child with autism who did not use verbal communication before participating in HEART but started to use words for the first time through the program. Another student, Davit,[3] experienced developmental delays but thrived under the personalized attention, targeted stress reduction techniques, and self-expression activities with his teachers. Over time, Davit gained confidence in his abilities and formed positive relationships with both peers and adults. His parents noticed that he was expressing himself more articulately and was more able to navigate social situations. Davit's experience also began to inspire other families in his community: When they saw how much progress he had made, more families in Tbilisi began requesting HEART in preschools, and the municipal preschool management agency sought to increase access to the program, creating a network of support for children like Davit and ultimately paving the way for more inclusive and supportive early childhood education in Georgia.

What Has HEART Meant for Teachers? The HEART program and the professional development that accompanies it have had a significant impact on preschool teachers in Georgia. Those participating in the 2021 evaluation reported that they were now paying more attention to children's individual needs and challenges and that their attitudes toward children with disabilities in particular had evolved (Save the Children, 2021a). The increased self-confidence felt by teachers and a more reflective approach to supporting their students have led to a more supportive classroom environment. Ultimately, 76% of teachers reported they were better able to manage their classroom, 65% reported that they could better help children to calm down, and 60% said that HEART gave them knowledge and skills for better inclusion and engagement of children with special educational needs (Save the Children, 2021a). Additionally, HEART also impacted how teachers interact with other adults: 38% reported improved communication with parents, 25% began cooperating with colleagues more effectively, and 51% began to care more about their own emotional state, which positively affected their work and personal life (Save the Children, 2021a).

One particularly passionate preschool teacher is Sopo, who works in Rustavi and was concerned about the lack of professional development opportunities in her community. Despite her commitment to providing quality education to the young minds in her care, she felt a growing concern that her knowledge and skills might not be sufficient to meet the evolving needs of her students. Determined to enhance her capabilities and create a better learning and emotionally secure environment for her students, Sopo eagerly took on the opportunity to undergo HEART training, which ultimately became a turning point in her career. The immediate impact of HEART training on Sopo's personal and professional growth was a fresh new perspective on preschool education, along with a practical toolbox of innovative teaching methods. As Sopo applied the HEART activities in her classroom, she witnessed a positive transformation in her students. The once passive and disengaged learners became active participants in their education, demonstrating increased curiosity and enthusiasm for learning. Sopo's ability to create an emotionally supportive, creative, stimulating, and interactive learning environment became a beacon for other educators in Rustavi—through sharing her experiences with her colleagues, her local advocacy helped the program to flourish in her school and town. Recognizing the positive outcomes among Sopo's students, the local education authorities acknowledged Sopo as an exemplary teacher. She became a preschool program design advisor in her hometown and was selected among a core group of teachers to be trained as a HEART trainer to help introduce the program to others. Sopo's journey with HEART not only elevated her professional standing but also instilled a newfound confidence in her abilities as an educator. She became a mentor to her peers, sharing her knowledge and experiences to inspire a culture of emotionally supportive continuous learning within the community. Sopo continues to be a HEART Champion in Rustavi. Her experiences serve as a testament to the profound impact that investing in teachers' growth and development can have on the entire community.

Conclusion

The early years of a child's life are some of the most important in determining future cognitive, social, emotional, and physical skills, and experiences during this period can severely impact children's future outcomes. For young children, play and arts-based therapeutic approaches allow them to explore, process, and start to address feelings and experiences they may not be able to verbalize. HEART is a comprehensive and adaptable approach that can be used by trained and supported nonclinical facilitators in formal and nonformal preschool situations. In the HEART model, young children physically create art and benefit from the resulting relaxation and getting "lost in the process" that come with these kinesthetic and sensory activities. Given their developmental stage, being able to express themselves through music, movement, and play helps them to verbalize memories, ideas, and emotions. The group-based approach of all facilitated activities and sharing circles at the end of the art-making process, gives space for intra- and interpersonal connection and social reflection. HEART promotes agency and choice, which is often lacking for many young children, especially those in crisis contexts.

Through the examples from development contexts in Mexico and Georgia and the humanitarian contexts in Nigeria and Tanzania, early childhood programming in HEART is focused mainly on preschool aged children and their teachers, CFS facilitators, and caregivers as appropriate. The program's focus on play, safe self-expression, and managing emotions improves well-being not only for children but also for the adults in their lives. Preliminary evaluation findings from the Mexico and Georgia programs have indicated positive results regarding children's emotional regulation and expression and improved well-being for parents, caregivers, and teachers. Feedback from preschool teachers and CFS facilitators in Tanzania and Nigeria points to improved attendance and increased confidence, empathy, and communication. The sustained and widespread adoption of HEART in Mexico and Georgia and the program's sustained support in refugee and IDP camps in Tanzania and Nigeria are indicative of how simple, adaptive, and developmentally appropriate interventions can transform the early childhood educational experience.

Key Takeaways

- Arts-based psychosocial support in early childhood settings can support the well-being of young children in ways that compensate for some of the negative impacts of adverse experiences.
- The experience of HEART in early childhood settings in different parts of the world offers important insights into cost-effective and sustainable methods for improving psychosocial well-being, learning, and development of young children.

Notes

1 Name changed for privacy.
2 Name changed for privacy.
3 Name changed for privacy.

Chapter 6

HEART in Childhood

Asli Arslanbek, Carolyn Alesbury, Dario Lipovac,
Miroslava Marjanovic, and Jean Nkhonjera

Introduction

Childhood and adolescence can be a time of great stress. For many children, exposure to continuous change, increasing responsibility, challenging family environments, high academic expectations, and/or increasingly complex social relationships can serve as significant stressors, depending on their individual circumstances (Siddique & D'Arcy, 1984; Spirito et al., 1991; Compas, Orosan, & Grant, 1993; Flinn & England, 1995; Fields & Prinz, 1997; Compas & Wagner, 2017). These stressors exist even during the "best of times" and can serve as compounding sources of anxiety during periods of instability.

For children exposed to unexpected and adverse events, such as natural disasters, pandemics, war, or armed conflict, the impact on their mental health can be far more significant, even leading to an increased risk of developing PTSD, anxiety, or depression (Kousky, 2016; Ng et al., 2015; Paardekooper, De Jong, & Hermanns, 1999; Reed et al., 2012). The memories of armed conflict and war can also resurface in communities long after the events have ended. For example, the arrival of new migrants or the outbreak of new violence can trigger painful war-related memories from individuals' pasts. Such events can also evoke transgenerational trauma in children born after the war, where the traumatic experiences of one generation are passed down to subsequent generations (Sarkissian & Sharkey, 2021). In cases of transgenerational trauma, children and grandchildren may find themselves experiencing symptoms or "reliving" certain aspects of the traumatic events endured by previous generations (Dikyurt, 2023).

Adverse situations are not necessarily startling or time-bound, however. Children can be exposed to ongoing stressors related to family economic pressure as well as to ongoing community health concerns. For example, children affected by HIV/AIDS may experience adverse effects on their mental health, stemming from the particular stigma and discrimination associated with HIV (U.S. Department of Health and Human Services; Betancourt et al., 2013), as well as limited access to health care, which tends to be more prevalent in rural

DOI: 10.4324/9781003367529-7

areas than in urban environments (Basta, Shacham, & Reece, 2009). For children who have lost one or both parents to HIV/AIDS, studies have found a direct link to increased feelings of anxiety, hopelessness, loneliness, and depression (Lata & Verma, 2013). This loss can also lead to behavioral problems, emotional detachment, and feelings of fear (Lata & Verma, 2013). Children who live with HIV positive parents and those who are HIV positive themselves have also been found to be more at risk of exposure to violence in their homes and communities, which in turn is associated with lower self-esteem and higher rates of depression and problem behaviors (Skeen et al., 2016). Many factors can affect the way children respond psychologically to a stressor or an adverse event. The severity of the situation, personality characteristics, individual coping styles, and the availability of social support and resources can impact a child's stress response and resiliency (Kovács et al., 2022; Neece, Green, & Baker, 2012; Terranova, Boxer, & Morris, 2009; Norris et al., 2002; Udwin et al., 2000; Tol et al., 2008; Paardekooper et al., 1999). Mental health services are crucial in helping children mitigate the stressors in their young lives. Unfortunately, access to professional services is extremely limited, with some countries experiencing a ratio of fewer than 0.5 psychiatrists for every 100,000 people (Kaku et al., 2022). Scaling up of mental health services for children and youth therefore requires the expansion of non-clinical psychosocial support services through trusted adults already present in the community. Through these individuals, emotionally supportive environments can be established to help children mitigate the impact of stressors and adverse events.

The Arts as a Protective Factor

Creative art therapies are reported as one of the most common mental health and psychosocial support intervention modalities used in post-conflict settings, especially with children and adolescents, and have been used regularly in response to a variety of emergencies (Chilcote, 2007; Kamali et al., 2020; Ugurlu, Akca, & Acarturk, 2017). Art in general can help children organize memories that were disrupted due to stressful or traumatic events, provide normalcy in a safe and predictable environment, and offer a rewarding experience that supports mastery (Berberian, 2019). Art also helps children see themselves as survivors rather than victims (Orr, 2007), renews their sense of purpose, brings comfort (Mohr, 2014), and supports problem-solving skills (Huss et al., 2016). Furthermore, making arts-based interventions available to teachers has been found to generate increased understanding of children's psychosocial needs and greater feelings of confidence in the classroom, indicating that such interventions can be beneficial for children both individually and with their relationships with their teachers (Furlager, 2018).

Use of the Arts in Cultural Practices in HEART

In various parts of the world, art is embedded in healing and protective rituals and has been used for community practices of well-being (Arslanbek, Malhotra, & Kaimal, 2022). In Malawi, dancing is a central cultural element that has a presence in the country's political culture, religious practices, and social life (Gilman, 2011, 2015). Not only dancing but also rhythm and singing are incorporated as healing elements in rituals. For example, a traditional Malawian practice, Vimbuza, which includes drumming, singing, and body movement (Gilman, 2015), is used as a healing ritual in the northern region of the country. Special HEART sessions in Malawi highlight this, and other local cultural arts traditions, by inviting children and local community members to share these activities in the schools and centers. In Uganda, indigenous dancing practices were suspended under British rule and began to reflourish after independence in 1962. Indigenous music and dance were introduced in curriculums in schools and in academic courses in university education, with an attempt to reintroduce indigenous knowledge to the community (Mabingo, 2020). The HEART program in Bosnia and Herzegovina also embraces traditional music and song, incorporating activities that involve participants singing traditional folk songs such as Sevdalinka. Such examples demonstrate how expressive artistic practices are accessible and embedded in community life across different countries and contexts and can be integrated into local HEART programming.

Integrating HEART in Primary and Secondary Schools

Despite the clear linkages between art and psychosocial well-being, far too few children have regular access to arts-based activities, in emergency settings or otherwise. Schools serve as a critical access point for arts-based mental health and well-being services for children because teachers and administrators are often the first to notice problematic symptoms, and schools can offer a safe, familiar environment for students to participate in support programs. Unfortunately, limitations on budget and time, as well as prioritization of more "rigorous" school subject matter such as reading and math, often lead arts-based activities to be less of a priority in schools and in teacher training programs (Gibson & Larson, 2007; Davies, 2010).

Recognizing the scheduling difficulties faced by teachers in formal primary and secondary schools, HEART is designed to be adapted to the specific time slots and platforms available. This approach includes being integrated directly into the curriculum, incorporated in weekly school programs, or delivered through separate after-school programs. For example, in contexts where teachers themselves are not able to integrate HEART into their time with students, school counselors have been able to take the lead on HEART activities with students outside of core instruction time. Likewise, in emergency contexts where schools are not yet able to restart, or integrating HEART into the school day is not possible, community centers offer an alternative platform for delivering HEART activities to primary- and secondary-school age children. These activities typically take place after school (or during the day if schools are not yet open) and are facilitated by trained paraprofessionals rather than by certified classroom teachers.

The intensity of HEART programming can vary as well, reaching children where and when they are available. Whereas the programming model is intended to be implemented across a full nine-month school year, it can be adapted to meet specific contextual programming needs. These needs sometimes include shorter implementation cycles of three to six months or launching as a condensed package in initial stages and then transitioning to the full program when feasible. The frequency and duration also shift not only across different responses, but sometimes within them. For example, HEART was initially launched in Eastern Ukraine in 2014 and was able to operate in stable long-term programming through classrooms, before shifting to a home support model during COVID-19 school closures in 2020 and 2021 and later being paused in early 2022 when new armed conflict caused schools to close. Later in 2022, it transitioned to an emergency approach, reaching children in shelters, and then in 2023 started to be used again in primary schools as children returned to school in areas where it was safe to do so and as of early 2024, expansion of HEART in primary schools continues across several regions of Ukraine.

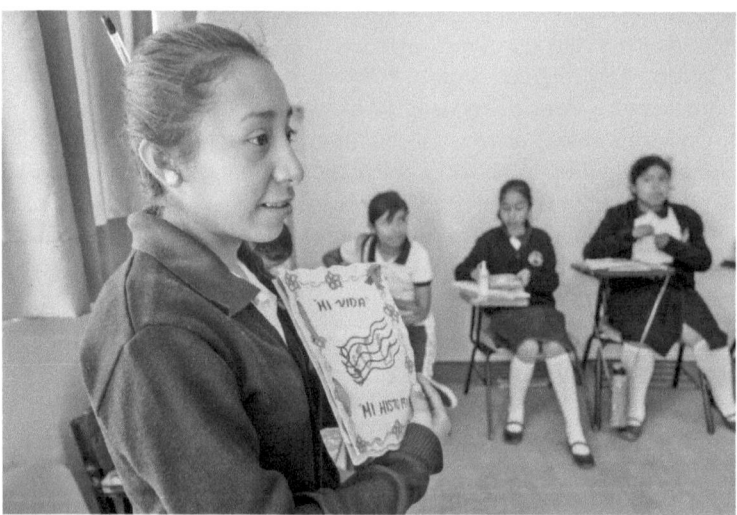

Figure 6.1 A child shares a book she created during a HEART session at her primary school in Mexico

Source: Save the Children

In addition to the mental health benefits of incorporating expressive arts into classrooms, some teachers have chosen to utilize arts-based approaches beyond their HEART sessions, by integrating their arts into their instructional approaches in the classroom. This approach can help to stimulate learning among diverse learners. The flexibility offered by incorporating different teaching approaches is well aligned with the Universal Design for Learning (UDL), which encourages variety in the way that students are presented with information, engaged in learning, and asked to demonstrate what they have understood (Rose & Meyer, 2002). By incorporating this variety into lesson design from the outset, teachers maximize the choices that students are able to make, improving the conditions for learning and achievement. Teachers who have been able to implement arts-based teaching methodologies into their instructional approach have reported that it contributes to an easier balancing between different teaching styles compared to the traditional academic lecture-based approach. Teachers also reported that incorporating arts-based teaching methodologies into classrooms that also include HEART sessions has helped prevent professional burnout as the overall learning environment has become more emotionally supportive and creatively interactive on a daily basis, making it not only a supportive learning environment for students but also a supportive work environment for teachers.

HEART Back to School: Supporting the Safe Return Back to Primary School After the COVID-19 Pandemic in Malawi

HEART has been implemented in the Zomba District of Southern Malawi since 2013. In addition to being a district with one of the highest prevalence rates of HIV in children and adults in Malawi (Nutor et al., 2020), Zomba is also prone to natural disasters such as floods, and the majority of the population lives below the poverty line. In order to reach school-aged children, HEART has been integrated into local community centers as after-school programs (known as Children's Corners) and on a small scale into health clinics, particularly the Nutrition Rehabilitation Units and Pediatric Wards in order to provide a continuum of psychosocial support to children who frequently transition between schools to local health clinics.[1]

The after-school HEART program supports children mostly age 6–15, most often with two HEART sessions per week as part of a comprehensive after-school program that also includes sports and recreation activities and additional learning activities such as a program aimed at supporting improved literacy. An interesting component of HEART in Malawi is the making of arts supplies from local resources. Because certain art materials are not readily available to purchase in rural areas of Malawi, the local HEART team makes modeling clay, paints, and paint brushes through a variety of locally available natural materials and runs workshops through which children and teachers learned to make their own arts supplies. The program has been strongly supported by the district government, the Department of Education, and the departments of Social Welfare, Child Affairs, and Disability, both for its positive impact on children and for its cost-effectiveness.

In 2020, the Ministry of Education closed public preschools, primary schools, and secondary schools for seven months as part of the national COVID-19 lockdown. This also meant the closure of the after-school HEART program for primary and secondary-school age children in Malawi. The school closures left thousands of children at home to follow remote classes and lessons, many of them without appropriate support from their parents/ caregivers and/or without technological equipment to fully follow the remote lessons. This situation led to students reporting that they felt disconnected and isolated, which added to the stressors influencing their socioemotional functioning and overall well-being (Save the Children, 2021b). School closures and wider negative impacts of the COVID-19 pandemic on communities also disrupted children's support systems, leaving them more vulnerable to various risks, such as lack of protection, poor health, or food insecurity (Save the Children, 2021b). Teachers also experienced increased levels of stress during this time as they facilitated remote learning for children and worked to provide for their own livelihoods within the new operational context. Following the reopening of schools, teachers found themselves responsible not only for traditional academic learning but also for the psychosocial well-being of both themselves and their students.

To meet the unique needs arising from the situation, the local HEART team supported the integration of a condensed version of HEART into the primary schools in the district. "HEART Back to School" constituted approximately 20% of the full program and was used specifically to address the challenges imposed by the COVID-19 pandemic, ensuring an emotionally supportive transition back to school in the months following lockdown and remote learning. The primary objective was to facilitate a smoother transition back to school for children by creating a more gentle, creative, interactive, fun, and supportive environment that helped them to process and recover from the stress of recent months. The goal of the gradual transition with HEART Back to School was also intended to help children improve their concentration and communication, to be better able to re-engage in the formal learning environment.

Using this new model, the Malawi HEART team scaled up their HEART Back to School program to support 57 primary schools in Zomba including 46,246 children in addition to the more than 24,000 children attending centers where the standard after-school HEART program had previously been established. Key COVID-19 prevention measures were observed, including wearing masks, limiting the sizes of group sessions, allocating art materials to individual children and discouraging sharing of arts materials, supporting frequent handwashing, and, where possible, conducting activities outside and with social distancing.

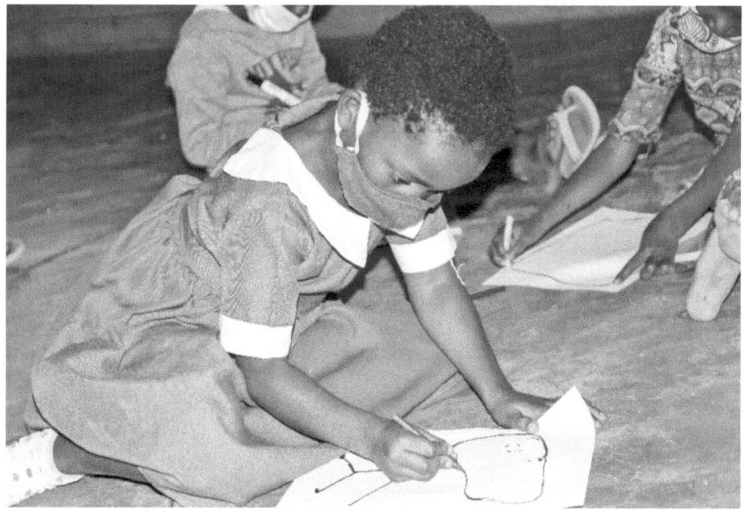

Figure 6.2 A child participates in HEART at her primary school in Malawi
Source: Save the Children

As HEART activities were made available to children during their return to school, they began to benefit from the opportunity to express themselves through creative and supportive communication. Peer-to-peer interactions began to improve (Save the Children, 2021b), and teachers began to note an impact on individual children including those that were previously socially withdrawn. Teachers and school counselors both reported that the HEART sessions played a significant role in boosting learner attendance and active participation in school. The play-based approach created more opportunities for children to have fun which served as additional motivation for student attendance. They noted observations of HEART activities fostering socialization, promoting emotional well-being, and supporting confidence building among children (Save the Children, 2021b). They felt that the HEART sessions helped children feel more at ease and comfortable when returning to school and reported that HEART's contribution to increased school attendance was also linked to teachers being better prepared to support children emotionally and respond to their needs.

Teachers also reported that they felt HEART helped improve teacher–learner relationships because they felt better able to relate to students beyond academic tasks. Teachers reported that students started interacting with their teachers more freely, including discussing social-emotional issues and obtaining referrals when needed. Some teachers even saw an impact beyond the classroom. As one teacher reported, "when I am chatting or interacting with family, community and peers, I employ HEART skills—which have become part of my daily living skills—to reduce the impact of negative emotions on me and others" (Save the Children, 2021b). Although the HEART Back to School program was initially intended for three months, to support the transition back to school after COVID-19 school closure, many teachers and school counselors continued with HEART sessions during the school day after the initial project period ended, and for students who no longer have access to HEART inside their school, they can attend the after-school HEART program in their local Children's Corners.

The use of the Condensed HEART Program in Malawi for a specific need at a specific time and place, with the option of sustaining or transitioning back to the regular local HEART programming model, is a useful example of the adaptability of HEART to meet changing local needs over time.

HEART Supporting South Sudanese and Democratic Republic of Congo Refugees in Uganda

Uganda hosts the largest refugee population in Africa and the third largest in the world, with a total of more than 1.5 million refugees, mainly from South Sudan, followed by the Democratic Republic of the Congo and Somalia, as of 2023 (European Commission, 2023; UNHCR, The UN Refugee Agency, 2023b). The country's supportive refugee policy environment—including the 2006 Refugee Act, the 2010 Refugee Regulations, and the 2017 Comprehensive Refugee Response Framework (CRRF)—allows refugees freedom of movement, access to education and health care, livelihood opportunities (land for farming and income generating), right to work, and access to national services.

Despite these protections, the refugee experience is harrowing, particularly for children, as they flee from conflicts and often reach Uganda exhausted, malnourished, distressed, and in need of health care. Children in many cases travel without their parents and are accompanied by other caregivers such as relatives and friends, which adds another layer of distress (Save the Children, 2022a). Although caregivers are typically a protective factor for children, they may be exhausted themselves by the severity of the violence experienced in the home country, the risks associated with displacement, the lack of social support, and the struggles to cope with their own stress from the experience (Bartolomei, Eckert, & Pittaway, 2013).

In Uganda, the HEART program has been carried out since 2016, focused initially in areas with high refugee populations in northern and western Uganda. In northern Uganda, the program is implemented in refugee settlements mainly for South Sudanese refugees and host communities, and in western Uganda in transit centers mainly for refugees from the Democratic Republic of the Congo. HEART has been integrated into community centers called Child Friendly Spaces (CFS), community-based child protection (CBCP) spaces, and alternative learning centers (ALS), working with children and youth. The goal of integrating HEART into educational and child protection emergency programming in Uganda is to address the psychological and socioemotional needs of children and complement other programming to support children's resilience, psychosocial well-being, and holistic development. As in Malawi, when certain art supplies are not available, they are created from local resources together with the community.

The integration of HEART into the monthly schedule of CFS serves as a valuable addition to the overall service provision, ensuring that children have access to structured and high-quality psychosocial support programs. Within the CFS environment, children regularly engage in HEART activities on a weekly basis. These activities encompass relaxation exercises, free arts, and structured activities, all facilitated by compassionate and well-trained adult facilitators. Considering that HEART is among the few available psychosocial support programs accessible to children, and acknowledging the significant psychological and socioemotional needs they possess, the children display a strong motivation to actively participate in the program on a regular basis. One of the major factors contributing to their enthusiasm is HEART's emphasis on play and expressive arts, incorporating local traditional games and artistic practices into the program.

Despite the program's ability to captivate children through its focus on the expressive arts, there are challenges. One of the main challenges is the 40:1 ratio of children to adult facilitators in most programming locations, which overwhelms not only the facilitators, but also the materials and the space itself. To accommodate this issue, facilitators split children into smaller, more manageable groups for scheduled HEART activities. Ultimately, the children have benefitted from the program, as evidenced by the fact that the facilitators consistently report improvements in the children's social skills, emotional regulation, expression of ideas, and participation as well as an overall decrease in conflict among children as they empathy, good listening skills, and become supportive of one another (Save the Children, 2021c; Save the Children, 2022a).

In 2021, the HEART program in Uganda was adapted through the response to the COVID-19 pandemic. Schools had been closed in the country twice; lockdown and travel restrictions had disrupted protective structures for children; and many students were distressed by their lack of progression in school. Economic stress at the family level also rose during the pandemic, impacting the type of support children were able to receive at home. During this time, HEART was rolled out in two phases. The first phase targeted the refugee settlements of Rwamwanja, Kyangwali, and Palorinya and focused on the procurement and distribution of art supplies to facilitate HEART activities at home. During the second phase, the program was extended to Kiryandongo and Yumbe, ultimately reaching 71% of Save the Children humanitarian operation areas in the country in addition to the development operational areas in Ntoroko, Bubdibugyo, and Kasese.

During this period, HEART facilitators, comprising primary school teachers, preschool teachers, alternative learning facilitators, and CFS facilitators, delivered a simplified version of the HEART program to children through home visits. Several significant challenges were encountered during this process including the scale of implementation because the number of HEART facilitators available was relatively small compared to the number of children who required support in their homes. This challenge was addressed by preparing and airing simple dramatic play-based relaxation activities via radio during the lockdown to supplement the home visits and strengthen the continuity of psychosocial support for children during a period of significant disruption in their young lives.

Once the COVID-19 restrictions lifted in Uganda, and children were able to return to their Child Friendly Spaces, community-based child protection spaces, and alternative learning centers, the HEART program transitioned back into its normal structure, with children attending face-to-face sessions with their facilitators in their normal program spaces.

HEART Adapting to Changing Needs in Bosnia and Herzegovina

Although the war in Bosnia and Herzegovina ended three decades ago, its legacy remains inescapable. European Union and North Atlantic Treaty Organization-led peacekeeping forces remain in the country as a reminder of the tenuous nature of peace and were recently doubled in response to the fragility of the current context. Further complicating the local situation is the continuous migration in and out of the country. As many Bosnians leave their homeland due to economic insecurity, others arrive. Over the past four years, tens of thousands of migrants and refugees have arrived in the country, most of whom have settled in Una-Sana Canton. Save the Children has been implementing HEART in Una-Sana Canton since 2016, when it was initially piloted as a regular activity in a number of primary schools. In 2018, Save the Children and the Ministry of Education, Science, Culture, and Sports of Una-Sana Canton signed a Memorandum of Understanding, whereby both groups committed to scaling the HEART program in all primary schools in the cantonal district. As part of the HEART scaling efforts, they agreed to establish three HEART resource centers each within one of three primary schools called HEART Friendly Schools, so that professionals from those schools could receive additional training and coaching to become supporters of neighboring schools.

As HEART programming expanded in primary schools across the cantonal district, feedback from the teachers and school counselors trained as HEART facilitators in the primary schools of Una-Sana Canton was extremely positive. For example, several teachers observed changes in more introverted children who were empowered by the activities to engage more with their classmates, with one teacher noting "children were so supportive towards each other that they inspired the involvement of introverted children in discussion, something that they have never done before" (Save the Children, 2019b). Others noted that students became more proactive and involved in other school activities after participating in HEART. Teachers also felt that they connected better with students, which can reinforce a positive school environment for students (Save the Children, 2019b). Many children described the HEART sessions as "their best class ever" and requested increased scheduling for more HEART sessions in their schools (Save the Children, 2019b). As student and teacher demand for HEART increased, so did scaling, to the extent where, as of 2024, HEART has been expanded to reach almost 60% of all primary school classrooms in the district.

Given the extent to which HEART had been institutionalized in Una-Sana Canton, in particular with the three HEART centers of excellence, the infrastructure was in place to expand the program to support refugee children as they arrived in the area. These children experienced significant stressors during their journey to Bosnia and Herzegovina. By the time they arrived in Una-Sana Canton, where the camps for migrants and refugees are located, they often presented in need of psychosocial support. In 2019, Save the Children, in collaboration with the Una-Sana Canton Ministry of Education, Science, Culture, and Sports, initiated HEART sessions as a component of a broader package of classes provided to refugee children, through four schools with dedicated

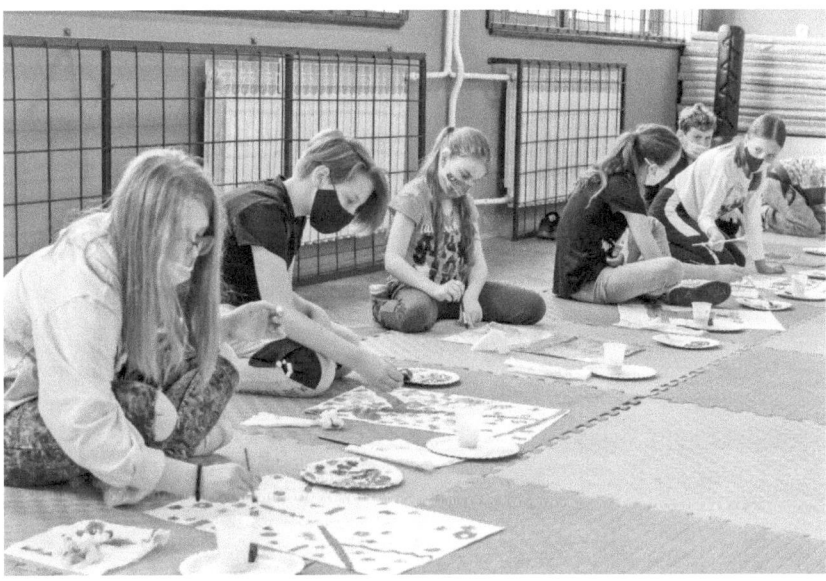

Figure 6.3 Children participate in HEART at their primary school in Bosnia and Herzegovina

Source: Save the Children

space for them, including the three schools originally established as centers for HEART excellence for the local HEART scaling partnership (the three original HEART Friendly Schools). These schools were specifically identified as creative and emotionally supportive locations where the integration of refugee learners could be prioritized. The refugee school support program was started in these schools to support refugee children to learn the Bosnian language, receive psychosocial support, socialize with other children, and get to know their teachers, so that they could eventually transition into the regular school system.

Language acquisition and adaptation to the school setting were the core focus of the refugee support program because most of the children did not have any school experience before arriving in Bosnia and Herzegovina. Through the HEART sessions, their social and emotional skills can be strengthened which helps to prepare them for the structured formal education environment. The use of HEART not only provided children with exposure to a structured school activity, but also assisted them in alleviating the stress associated with their transition into formal schooling.

The HEART facilitators involved in the refugee learner support program noted marked improvements in children's communication and adjustment to the learning environment. For example, many children who begin their formal education in the refugee school support program in Una Sana Canton have been able to transition to the regular school program after only a few months of language classes, HEART, and social activities with other children. Because the children attending the refugee support program transition into regular school classes after completing the preparatory program, they continue to participate in HEART because HEART has been fully scaled in all four of the primary schools selected for the refugee support program. This means that HEART is not only part of the process of transitioning into formal primary school education, but also a source of continued support on a weekly basis throughout the school year, providing a continuum of support for the refugee students throughout their school experience in Una-Sana Canton.

The HEART program continues to serve migrant and refugee children in Bosnia and Herzegovina as well as other members of the local community, as HEART scaling continues throughout Una-Sana Canton. More information about the scaling of HEART in primary schools in Bosnia and Herzegovina is provided in Chapter 10.

Discussion

Applying the HEART program within educational institutions is not only a viable approach but one that has demonstrated numerous advantages for students, teachers, and their interpersonal dynamics. In addition to helping teachers plan more effective lessons, HEART also shifts the overall atmosphere of the classroom by transferring the focus from the product of an activity to the process. During HEART, teachers prioritize patience in listening, being non-judgmental, and showing compassion, and do not assign grades or scores to students. The experiences in Malawi, Uganda, and Bosnia and Herzegovina have shown that classrooms that incorporate these behaviors can lead to less isolation and better group cohesion as well as provide a departure from the traditional one-sided, linear approach to teaching. In addition to addressing student socioemotional well-being, HEART also helps create an environment conducive to improved student-learning outcomes.

The examples detailed above also showcase the adaptability and versatility of the HEART program. Through incorporating local art traditions and adjusting the frequency and volume of activities to meet the needs of a specific context, the program is implementable across the full spectrum of the long-term development of programming to a short-term humanitarian response.

Conclusion

School-aged children are exposed to a variety of stressors throughout their young lives. In this post-COVID-19 world, all have lived through a pandemic, and many others have also been impacted by violence, war, and natural disasters. All of these issues are in addition to the academic, social, and family stresses that children must balance on a daily basis. Managing these stresses is a key prerequisite to learning and developing. Children cannot be expected to thrive in school if they are grappling with intense stress. School has long been recognized as a safe, stable, and effective environment in which children can be provided with key services. Many teachers are eager to provide psychosocial support to their students but lack the training or flexibility of schedule to be able to do so effectively. HEART has been designed to help fill these gaps, in the time and space available to students—whether that is during lessons, in between classes, or at home. Experiences from Malawi, Uganda, and Bosnia and Herzegovina present key examples of how HEART has been successfully rolled out to school-aged children in a variety of contexts.

Key Takeaways

- HEART for school-aged children and youth provides a scalable approach to delivering psychosocial support to children who might not otherwise have access to services.
- In some areas, such as Una-Sana Canton in Bosnia and Herzegovina, the local government has taken steps to institutionalize the HEART program within their broader education system.
- Although HEART is designed to provide stress relief and psychosocial support, there are clear benefits for student-learning outcomes as children

become more comfortable in the school and their teachers become more comfortable varying their teaching methods.

- The HEART program is adaptable to development and humanitarian contexts and has been used across the full range of the global program spectrum.

Note

1 Children affected by HIV/AIDS, malaria, and/or malnutrition can spend weeks or months receiving treatment in health clinics each year. Providing HEART in both their after-school programs and their local health clinics ensures that such children receive consistent psychosocial support throughout the year because their access to the program does not end during periods of hospitalization.

Chapter 7

"We Are Alike Now"

HEART for All Children

Carolyn Alesbury, Aida Bekic, and Ana Lagidze

What has this meant for Natia?

When describing a program, it is easy to get lost in the high-level details about total children reached and activities delivered. Equally important, however, are the individual experiences of children and families who participated in the program. Therefore, we would like to begin this chapter with Natia. Natia is a 5-year-old girl living in Georgia who absolutely loves participating in the HEART for All program. She likes to replicate activities she has learned at her preschool when she returns home, and is eager to tell her brother and sister about what she does each day. When her cousins come to visit, she suggests shifting their usual play to arts-based activities instead. Natia's mother has noticed some key changes in her daughter since joining HEART for All. Natia used to find it difficult to build relationships and interact with strangers. She has spastic diplegia cerebral palsy, which impacts both her fine and gross motor skills. Her mother says that Natia's ability to hold a pencil or brush in her hand has improved through the program, and in addition to strengthened motor skills, she is also better able to express and perceive emotions. She is more relaxed and sociable and more able to adapt to the environment around her. Natia's participation in HEART has not only helped her build physical and social emotional skills but has also given her the opportunity to interact with her peers in new ways. According to her teacher, Natia was delighted by a particular HEART relaxation activity that involved everyone crawling on the floor together—she turned to her mother and said : "look Mom, the children are walking like me. We are alike now."

DOI: 10.4324/9781003367529-8

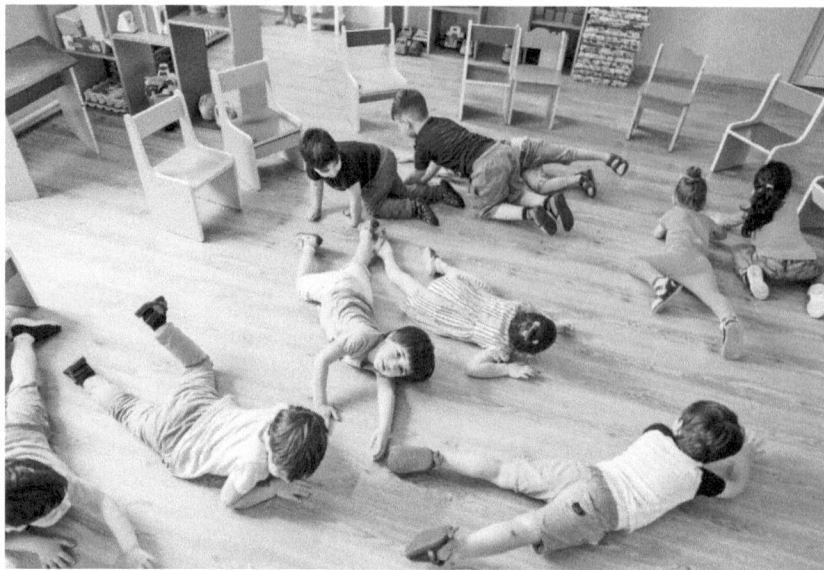

Figure 7.1 A HEART activity that uses dramatic play to promote relaxation at a preschool in Georgia

Source: Save the Children

Identifying a Gap

As the HEART program expanded in the early 2010s, it began reaching more children across a range of countries and contexts. The children participating in HEART represented a cross-section of those typically enrolled in schools, preschools, and CFS in each area, including some children with disabilities. Although the initial HEART guidance did not provide specific tools or tips for meeting the needs of children with disabilities, some facilitators began making accommodations on their own, and anecdotes from their positive experiences soon spread across the global team.

The psychosocial benefits from these early examples were undeniable. In the West Bank, a Palestinian preschool student with a physical disability went from having difficulty socializing with her peers to engaging and interacting happily with classmates through HEART activities. At a refugee camp in Jordan, a Syrian preschool student who was previously not willing to wear his prescribed eyeglasses finally felt comfortable doing so after his teacher led the entire class in an adapted HEART activity that involved creating, decorating, and wearing paper glasses and talking about differences, so that he was no longer a target for bullying.

These stories highlighted the importance of inclusive psychosocial support programming for children with disabilities and identified a key gap in the HEART materials—the absence of specific guidance on accommodating children with disabilities. The extent to which HEART activities were inclusive of all children depended entirely on the will and expertise of individual facilitators. Addressing this gap would require targeted action to ensure that all facilitators had access to the guidance they needed to meaningfully include children with disabilities in HEART programming and provide them with psychosocial support (PSS) alongside their peers.

In the education sector, Save the Children has extensive experience including children with disabilities, from its flagship Student Needs Action Pack, which guides teachers through pedagogical accommodations to support the needs of children with mild to moderate disabilities, to more extensive workforce developmental interventions that provide specialized services to children with more severe disabilities. Drawing on these internal resources, the team worked with local organizations for persons with disabilities to create a version of HEART that could more intentionally include children with any type of disability. In HEART for All and in this chapter, we apply the United Nations Convention on the Rights of Persons with Disabilities definition of disability, which is "those who have long-term physical, mental, intellectual or sensory impairments which in interaction with various barriers may hinder their full and effective participation in society on an equal basis with others" (UNCRPD, Article 1). In the areas where HEART for All was piloted, this most often included children with physical or motor challenges, difficulty seeing and/or hearing, difficulties with learning or behavior, difficulties communicating or interacting with others, or sensory difficulties.

Research Base: Psychosocial Support for Children with Disabilities

Barriers and Stressors

Research about children with disabilities is inherently challenging because the definition of disability can fluctuate across contexts, screening programs are not universally accessible, and stigma can influence the answers individuals provide to questions linked to disability. Estimates on the percentage of children with disabilities therefore vary considerably across countries, from 1% in North Korea, to 27% in the Central African Republic (UNICEF, 2021). Prevalence is also known to increase during times of armed conflict and crisis: For example, currently, an estimated 28% of Syria's population has a disability, which is nearly twice as high as the average global prevalence rate (UN HNAP Syria, 2021). At the global level, these percentages equate to hundreds of millions of children, an estimated nearly 240 million worldwide (UNICEF, 2021), making their inclusion a relevant consideration for every community in every country. However, despite the scale of students affected, children with disabilities face significant barriers to participating in society alongside their peers and are less likely to be included in educational and early stimulation programs (UNICEF, 2021).

The need for psychosocial support for children with disabilities is significant because the prevalence of mental health difficulties tends to be higher than average among people with disabilities. A study of over 4,000 children in an early childhood program in Australia found that, whereas students without disabilities have a one in eight chance of experiencing mental health problems, the odds increase to one in three among children with disabilities, and one in two for children with multiple disabilities (Dix et al, 2010). This trend carries across different types of disabilities, with evidence of increased rates of depression among students with learning disabilities, hearing loss, reduced vision, and epilepsy (McMillan and Jarvis, 2013). Parents of children with autism spectrum disorder (ASD) also report that their child experiences anxiety at nearly eight times the rate of parents of children without ASD, according to a study of more than 62,000 American children and youth (Kerns et al., 2017). Even for children without depression or other documented mental health difficulties, psychosocial well-being is impacted both directly and indirectly by barriers linked to the child's disability. Directly, some children's disabilities (and the inability of their educational experiences to accommodate them) may impact their development of key social emotional competencies, such as self-regulation and social and emotional skills (Westwood, 2011). Indirectly, students who are struggling in class or who face an inflexible teacher with low expectations may have a harder time developing self-efficacy, resilience, and problem-solving skills (Westwood, 2011; Jarvis, 2011). These issues can also make them more susceptible to the impacts of high levels of stress after emergencies (Mann et al., 2021). Compounding all of these concerns, students with disabilities are also at increased risk of being bullied by their peers, which itself can lead to depression and anxiety. A study of more than 100 students with disabilities aged 8–17 in the United States found that the strongest predictors of increased depression or anxiety were bullying and ostracism (American Academy of Pediatrics, 2012). This problem is far reaching: UNICEF estimates that, worldwide, children with disabilities are 41% more likely to feel discriminated against, and 51% more likely to report feeling unhappy than their peers without disabilities (UNICEF, 2021).

Stressors for children with disabilities are also not limited to negative interactions that take place in school. In fact, studies show that home environments themselves can be extremely stressful, not only for children with disabilities but for their parents and their siblings as well. Parents of children with disabilities are often more stressed than parents of children without disabilities, a situation that is linked to direct factors such as the child's challenging behavior, as well as indirect factors such as a lack of financial resources, services, and support systems (Hsiao, 2018; Gupta and Singhal, 2005). This parental stress then influences their parenting approaches and the type and extent of emotional support they are able to provide their children, which in turn influences the child's own social emotional development (Hsiao, 2018; Gupta and Singhal, 2005). Siblings of children with disabilities are also exposed to these patterns and can experience feelings of unbalanced attention from parents, which can generate depression, anger, embarrassment, guilt, and loneliness (Gupta and Singhal, 2005). Ultimately, these factors can combine and reinforce each other to create home environments with high levels of psychosocial distress among multiple family members.

Benefits of Psychosocial Support

Evidence shows that when there is no targeted intervention, social and behavioral challenges are likely to continue throughout a child's education and lead to poor learning and mental health outcomes. A longitudinal study of more than 500 students in the United States found that students who demonstrated behavioral and academic problems in first grade had negative school and social outcomes by 12th grade, highlighting the strong link between behavior and academic skills/outcomes (Darney et al., 2013). However, despite recognition of the importance of supporting these children, children with disabilities are often missed by community-level psychosocial support programs (among other services). This situation is especially prevalent in times of emergency or uncertainty, when social services are further disrupted or reduced.

A systematic study of psychosocial support services provided to Syrian refugees found that although "refugees with disabilities are the most vulnerable and invisible group of refugees and asylum seekers" (Alodat, Alshagran, & Al-Bakkar, 2021, p. 1), provision of specialized PSS services to meet their needs remains a major gap. Core guiding documents, such as the Inter-Agency Standing Committee (IASC) Guidelines on Mental Health and Psychosocial Support in Emergency Settings, indicate that people with disabilities should be included in programs (IASC, 2007), but practical guidance on how to do so, particularly for children with disabilities, has lagged behind. As a promising recent step, the IASC released a new Information Note on Disability and Inclusion in MHPSS in 2024 (IASC, 2024).

PSS programming for children with disabilities not only provides support to the children themselves but has the potential to benefit their families, because studies have shown that support systems and trust in interventions can actually help lower parental stress (Hastings and Johnson, 2001). The value of arts-based programming specifically in enhancing the social and emotional well-being of children with disabilities is extensive. Providing the opportunity for students to participate in structured arts activities with their peers can establish an inclusive and manageable environment for children to engage and practice their social skills, something that is particularly important for children with ASD (Gabriels, 2003). A study of 44 students with ASD participating in expressive arts and group therapy in the United States found improved social skills among students as reported by teachers and parents, with improvement across all measured domains of social skills, including statistically significant improvement in terms of assertion, internalizing behaviors, hyperactivity, and problem behavior (Epp, 2008). Benefits have been observed for children with other types of disabilities as well. A study of 93 Israeli students with learning disabilities found that children who participated in art therapy programming demonstrated better adjustment than their peers who only received academic support, as measured by a child behavior checklist (Freilich and Shechtman, 2010). Additionally, a study of six children with intellectual disabilities in India found that across the duration of their participation in arts-based therapy, the children demonstrated steady improvement in core skill areas, including attention, group interaction, and expression (Thergaonkar & Daniel, 2019).

Psychosocial support and the benefits of arts-based therapeutic programs for children with disabilities remain understudied areas. Results from studies that do exist are not always comparable because they track different outcome measures across different groups of children who participate in different types of arts programs. However, the data that do exist, combined with the positive anecdotal evidence from early HEART programming and more recent qualitative findings after the rollout of HEART for All, more than justify the continued expansion of the HEART program to actively support children with disabilities across the globe.

HEART for All

Adaptation

The development of HEART for All began in 2016 with the establishment of a cross-country team of experts in HEART, education, and inclusion of children with disabilities. Based on organizational experience implementing inclusive educational programming, key priorities for the adaptation were identified.

First, the team acknowledged that there is no such thing as "activities for children with disabilities." The spectrum of disability is wide and complex, and activities that some children with disabilities can complete are not the same activities that other children with disabilities can complete. Likewise, activities that are "not designed" specifically for children with disabilities may still be perfectly accessible for some children. The team, therefore, sought not to develop a separate package of HEART activities but rather to provide guidance for facilitators on how to adapt HEART activities based on the specific identified needs of individual children in their programs.

Second, recognizing that in most contexts where Save the Children operates, many children do not have a formal diagnosis of disability. Therefore, the team planned to focus guidance on the *functional challenges* children experience rather than on specific labels or diagnoses. This choice is a practical one, given that many facilitators do not have access to formal diagnoses of their students and an ethical one, because introducing labels into a context where a professional diagnosis is not possible can lead to mislabeling and increased stigma. Members of the task team had experienced this firsthand in previous projects, where teachers estimated that a large (and statistically unlikely) portion of their students must have dyslexia because they were not learning to read quickly. Keeping the focus on identifying and addressing students' functional challenges also aims to steer the facilitator toward selecting suggested accommodations that are merited by the individual profile of the student rather than by a label associated with that student. Using this approach effectively requires that the facilitators get to know each child as an individual and use open communication with the child and their caregiver(s) to consistently monitor and update accommodations as needed. Effectively including children with disabilities is not an on/off switch and is unlikely to be something accomplished immediately and without adjustments. It is important for implementers to be prepared to try multiple approaches and adapt with the child in order to maximize their efforts.

Third, the team recognized that inclusion is not something that starts and ends in the HEART classroom. True inclusion requires steps to be taken well before the HEART sessions are scheduled to ensure that all children are proactively included and welcomed. It also requires consistent messaging, accommodation, and demonstration that the needs of individual students will be met in order for them to feel truly supported to attend the session.

With the common understanding and agreement in these key areas, volunteers on the team from Georgia, Armenia, Bosnia and Herzegovina, and the United States worked together to develop the first draft of a HEART for All guidance note. The guide included information on the rights background underpinning the approach, step-by-step instruction for facilitators on incorporating inclusion throughout the cycle of their program activities, and targeted guidance on accommodations and assistive technology designed to meet the needs of children with specific types of functional challenges. Based on feedback from organizations for persons with disabilities and implementers on the most common types of disabilities they encountered in their programs, the guidance document prioritized seven key areas of functional challenge:

- Physical or motor challenges
- Difficulty seeing

- Difficulty hearing
- Difficulty learning or understanding
- Difficulty staying focused and "well-behaved"[1]
- Hypersensitivity or hyposensitivity
- Difficulty communicating
- Difficulty with social interaction

Initial pilot trainings took place in Armenia and Albania, with the program soon expanding to Georgia, Bosnia and Herzegovina, and Kosovo. These first five Save the Children offices implemented a regional program for children with disabilities and incorporated the HEART for All activities seamlessly into their approach. This initial launch was followed by separate programs in Malawi and Mexico, as well as ongoing continued expansion to additional country contexts. Detailed examples from some of these HEART for All implementation locations are provided in the case stories below.

Cross-Country Findings and Reflections

Through the Eastern European regional project *Community-Based Services for Children with Disabilities*, Save the Children worked with local partners in Armenia, Georgia, Albania, Bosnia and Herzegovina, and Kosovo to establish comprehensive and sustainable community centers that provided critical services to children with disabilities and their families, including physical therapy, occupational therapy, and psychosocial support. Among the services provided through these centers, psychosocial support initially posed the biggest challenge due to the insufficient availability of mental health services in the region and the lack of disability-inclusive PSS programs in the countries where the project was implemented. Understanding that continuous participation of children in HEART activities can lead to more confident and secure individuals, all five countries in the program incorporated HEART for All into their community centers, serving as a robust cross-country pilot of the new guidance. The multifunctional nature of the community centers meant that adults trained to implement HEART included non-formal educators, psychologists, physiotherapists, special education teachers, and support staff.

The final evaluation of the regional project found that HEART brought practitioners and children together into an arts-based interactive setting that previously did not exist. This venue included the use of HEART in self-help groups and mixed-ability social groups, which strengthened opportunities for socialization and inclusion and boosted children's confidence. Children were reported to be better able to express their feelings, communicate effectively and willingly with adults and peers, and discover new artistic skills that contributed to self-expression and unlocked creativity (Save the Children, 2019a). Although

HEART was introduced primarily as a psychosocial support program, it was also found to be beneficial for development and creative learning; specifically, some components of the program addressed certain occupational therapy goals, such as improving fine motor skills (Raskovic, Obradovic, & Koprivica, 2019).

Anecdotally, facilitators noted that since participating in the activities, children demonstrated increased self-confidence and ability to recognize and communicate their feelings, share memories, and regulate emotions and behavior, as well as increased socialization and cooperation with their peers. Children also displayed improvement in key areas of development, such as motor skills, concentration, decision making, and math and language skills, in addition to an ability to more effectively cope with stressful situations. Benefits also extended to positive changes in the perceptions of adults. For example, the facilitators demonstrated more open and optimistic attitudes, including the following:

1. Adults must be adaptive and flexible to meet the diverse needs of the students they support, including children with disabilities.
2. There are many difficulties that can be easily and affordably addressed through simple accommodations.
3. Sometimes traditional teaching methods themselves are the biggest obstacles to disability inclusion.

These important shifts in thinking can lead to the establishment of a more trusting environment, which in turn supports children's cognitive development and increases adults' expectations, further improving their relationships with each other.

With this initial positive feedback, the HEART for All program was recognized as an approach that could be useful in settings outside of the community-based centers. As a result, the teams in Armenia, Albania, Georgia, and Kosovo all started implementing it through other sectors and programs, including new programming in preschools, primary schools, and community centers for children and youth. The team in Armenia named HEART as one of the most unintended positive impacts of the project. Ultimately, the program was so successful that it was integrated into the formal framework documented in the project publication "Supporting Inclusion of Children with Disabilities: Model of Community-Based Services" (Raskovic, Obradovic, & Koprivica, 2019).

Case Stories

The case stories that follow were selected to show a cross-section of HEART for All in different regions, settings, and approaches. Two of the examples (Albania and Georgia) came from the initial pilot program through community-based services for children with disabilities, whereas the other two examples show how the program has been replicated in informal (Malawi) and formal (Mexico) educational facilities.

Albania

HEART for All was rolled out in Albania in early 2017 through community-based centers for children with disabilities that had been established in Durres and Vlore the prior year. Psychosocial support, despite being recognized as essential for the overall developmental success of children, posed an initial challenge in the community-based centers, because programs of this type that are accessible to children with disabilities are very rare in Albania. The unique niche filled by HEART for All, as well as the enthusiasm of the centers' occupational therapists to introduce expressive arts activities, led to the adoption of the program in both centers. A total of eight staff members from the two centers participated in the initial training, which ultimately led to 33 children benefiting from HEART for All in the first year, including children with cerebral palsy, Down syndrome, autism spectrum disorder, and developmental delays, among other types of physical, intellectual, and multiple disabilities. General impressions of the HEART facilitators working with children were positive. They observed that children immensely enjoyed engaging in the arts activities at their own pace and style.

The biggest initial challenge was that many of these children could not maintain their focus or remain calm throughout an entire activity. They were very easily agitated by their peers as a consequence of being either isolated or bullied for their disability in their past. Previously, teachers rarely showed patience or appreciation for their work, which center staff reported as a key change and success factor in the implementation of HEART for All. Over time, through careful exposure and engagement, children were observed participating in the program with increased self-esteem, engagement, and visible joy, as well as effectively communicating and collaborating with other children.

Facilitators of HEART for All also observed changes in themselves. They reported that they became more empathetic, patient, and skilled in regulating different challenging behaviors with children, which in turn modeled empathy, calmness, and respectfulness back to the children. Parents as well reported positive experiences. The mother of Arben, a child with cerebral palsy, who had many difficulties moving, playing, and communicating, noted that HEART provided her son with an opportunity to develop his fine and gross motor skills and his cognitive skills (particularly thinking and reasoning) and to significantly improve his self-esteem, self-expression, and attention for learning. Together with his peers at the center, Arben participated in many group activities and was able to coordinate and collaborate, often assisting his peers with group activities. After activities finished, he was able to share his artwork, his favorite parts of the process, and express his

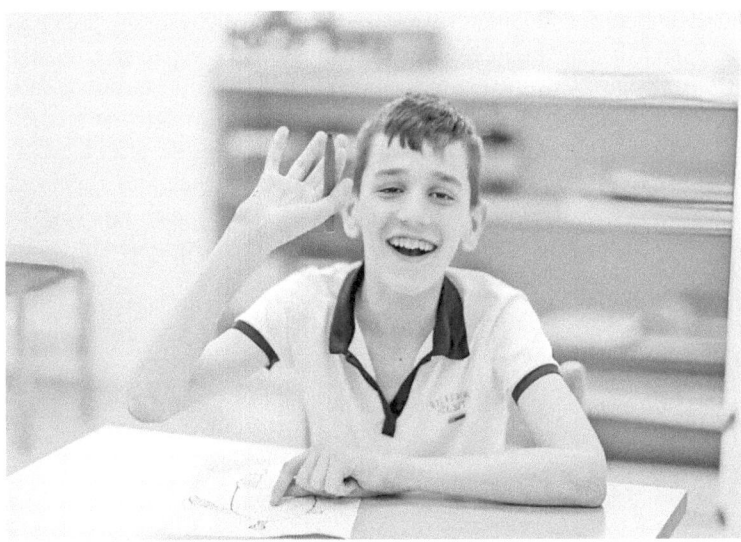

Figure 7.2 Arben participates in HEART at his support center in Albania
Source: Save the Children

experience of certain emotions. His mother shared that through her son's art-work, she was able to develop a deeper understanding of his feelings and what made him angry, sad, or happy. Through HEART for All, Arben changed significantly. He was no longer silent and withdrawn, he smiled much more frequently both at home and at the center, and he seemed to enjoy his time in the center much more, especially during activities that facilitated socialization with his friends. After his first year participating in HEART, center staff noticed that his math and literacy skills improved and referred him for more complex support and rehabilitation services. As his mother put it, "Arben has changed, because he never went to school before and he missed so many things in his first 15 years. Here at the center, he became part of a group of friends—something he wanted so much."

After the initial year of implementation, Save the Children established another Community-Based Services (CBS) center for children with disabilities in Kukes Municipality in Albania and started gradually expanding and integrating the HEART program in other sectors. The community-based centers are now sustained and operated by local municipal governments. Ultimately, the positive feedback on HEART for All led to it being expanded to preschools and primary schools, particularly those focused on enabling and enhancing the inclusion of marginalized children, such as Roma and refugee children, as well as children with disabilities. Eventually the program was also expanded into social work programs, supporting children in residential care facilities during the deinstitutionalization and residential care transformation process in Albania. In 2019, the Ministry of Education of Albania accredited HEART as an in-service training option for the continued professional development of primary and secondary school teachers. This endorsement of HEART was re-issued after the COVID-19 lockdown to encourage teachers to continue to focus their professional development on psychosocial support and social emotional learning. This formal endorsement of the program has enabled its continued expansion in the education sector in Albania.

Georgia

In partnership with Association Anika, a leading Organization of Persons with Disabilities in Georgia, Save the Children rolled out HEART for All in 2018 through the Anika Day Care Center in Tbilisi and later in 2019, through a second center in Bolnisi. Both centers continue implementing HEART today, having reached approximately 275 children aged 6–18 over the last five years.

Prior to the integration of HEART for All, most of the activities and services within the centers were completed one-on-one or in small groups as specialist support sessions (for example, as physical therapy sessions or occupational therapy sessions). Interaction between center staff and children was limited to specialized care, and children had few opportunities within the center to interact

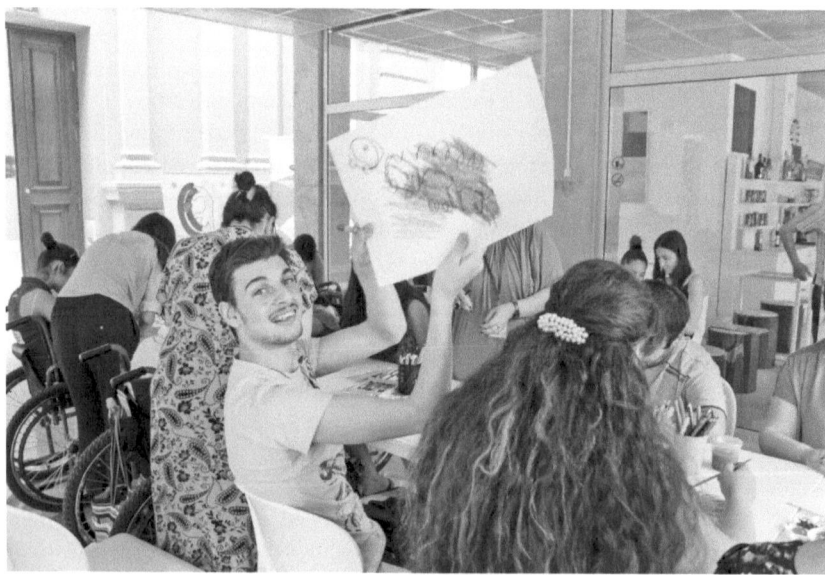

Figure 7.3 Youth participate in a HEART session at a support center in Georgia
Source: Save the Children

with each other and engage in group play. Further complicating the situation was the children's limited social interaction and behavior management skills, which often generated frustrations among children that facilitators were not easily able to mitigate.

After attending their first training for HEART for All and receiving arts supplies to support HEART activities in the centers, the Anika facilitators started to try two new approaches. The approaches included individual practitioners (such as speech therapists or physical therapists) incorporating arts-based activities in their one-on-one sessions with children as well as center practitioners organizing and co-facilitating group HEART activities for children. The center staff reported positive experiences with both approaches. Using arts methods in individual support sessions proved to be more interesting and engaging for the children, and the opportunity to participate in group HEART activities was a new experience that provided children with opportunities to socialize, play, communicate, and make new friends.

A significant piece of learning from the first phase of group HEART activities in the center was the experience of grouping children of different ages and different abilities together during activities. This change allowed children to utilize their skills to support each other. For example, children with mobility restrictions were supported by children without mobility restrictions. Children with difficulty seeing were supported by children with clear vision. Being able to use their abilities to help each other served to support coordination, communication, and self-confidence. For children who were often labeled by the

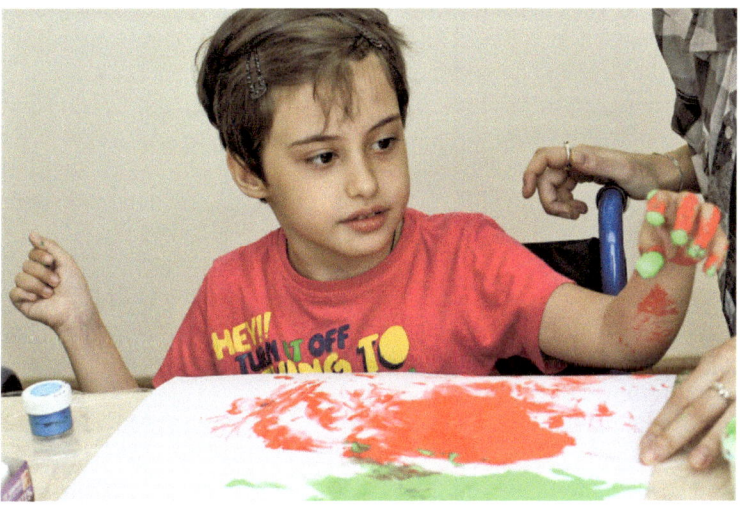

Figure 7.4 A child participates in HEART at a support center in Georgia

Source: Save the Children

functional challenges they experienced, the focus was now on their complementary strengths and abilities.

After several months of HEART implementation, center staff reported improved physical development, learning, and emotional regulation among the children in their care, and highlighted the way the arts activities supported fine and gross motor skills. Children demonstrated stronger skills in expressing themselves and in communicating with each other, both visually and verbally. Facilitators also recognized that the group activity process helped to build trusting relationships not only between children, but also between children and the staff. "It's like having a 'magic stick' that can immediately change the situation for engaging, fun and meaningful interaction with us and their peers," described one staff member. Over time, these positive experiences and relationships led to increased collaboration on HEART: For example, individual practitioners who previously provided individual support to specific children were now regularly co-facilitating group activities, which made the center a more creative, playful, emotionally understanding, and supportive place for everyone.

After the success of HEART for All in the day care centers, HEART was expanded to preschools in Georgia, ultimately reaching 30,000 children (5,147 with disabilities) across 155 preschools in Tbilisi, 22 preschools in Rustavi, and 37 in Kutaisi. By the end of 2023, a total of 755 adult facilitators had been trained to implement HEART for All with children in Georgia. Feedback from preschools teachers was similarly positive to that of the centers. Teachers reported improved professional skills and increased confidence in working with children with disabilities. They also reported a dramatic change in attitudes and practices toward teaching children with disabilities (among themselves and other staff in the preschools). A survey of preschool teachers trained on HEART for All in Georgia found that 76% felt that they were better able to manage their group after starting HEART for All in their classrooms. These shifts have also led to teachers more easily identifying children's individual challenges and ultimately planning and adapting other classroom activities to better meet their needs. The improvements have had a cascading effect on teacher motivation both within and beyond HEART, with one teacher sharing that she felt newly motivated and "for the first time, in a long time, I wanted to work more and more."

Beyond the overall group impact discussed previously, teachers also highlighted the observed impact with individual children, including significant changes in emotional regulation, behavior, and engagement in the classroom. One child with ASD began working with peers and using verbal communication for the first time in three years, while another child who was extremely reserved began using words for communication during her first HEART for All activity. Ultimately, the opportunity to express their emotions and opinions more freely has increased the independence of children with disabilities, which one teacher remarks helps them be "more open with both adults and each other, adapt to new situations, and express themselves in much more creative ways."

Malawi

Malawi, a country with a rich history of arts and music, has been contextualizing and adapting the HEART program for more than a decade. The program is delivered through Community-Based Childcare Centers (CBCCs), Children's Corners (after-school centers), primary schools, nutrition rehabilitation centers, and homes, to promote the psychosocial well-being of children affected by multiple adversities. After years of isolated positive experiences integrating children with disabilities into classrooms and centers through the HEART program, the team found that most children with disabilities were not fully participating in CBCC sessions or school-based programs because service providers, parents, community members, and teachers did not have the skills or awareness to effectively include them. Accordingly, the team decided to formally launch HEART for All in both CBCCs and Children's Corners in the Zomba District in southern Malawi. This act was complimented by Save the Children's Student Needs Action Pack approach in schools, which trains teachers to adapt their pedagogical approaches to meet the needs of different learners, including learners with disabilities.

Targeting preschool children in CBCCs and school-aged students in Children's Corners, the initial HEART for All training equipped staff, government partners, and CBCC/Children's Corner facilitators to deliver the program activities to children. The facilitators selected for this training had previously implemented the core HEART program and, after being trained on the new HEART for All adaptation, successfully rolled out the program in 232 CBCCs and 232 Children's Corners. Feedback from the facilitators indicated that after the introduction of HEART for All, they experienced increased attendance and participation from all children, regardless of the nature of their disability as well as increased new enrollment of children with identified disabilities, including 14 children with disabilities (five boys and nine girls) who had previously dropped out of school and re-enrolled to participate in HEART for All. HEART facilitators also worked with parents of children with disabilities and teachers to strengthen individualized and home support for some students. The facilitators reported observed improvements in both social emotional well-being and overall learning among children with disabilities, both as a result of increased attendance and participation in the centers (including and in addition to HEART) and the overall benefit of participating in HEART.

One child who was particularly impacted by the program was Joseph, who by the age of four was neither walking nor speaking, and would stand only with difficulty, which severely limited his ability to interact with his peers at the CBCC. As the CBCC caregivers began implementing HEART activities, they found that Joseph connected the most with movement and dance, and he began to move in his seat and showed more interest in his surroundings. He was also able to practice his fine motor skills through painting and drawing. Although he was not able to express his feelings and ideas audibly, he appeared to be more comfortable participating in arts activities. The patience of his teachers, and the emotional and social support that Joseph was exposed to through the program led to significant growth. After a few months, he was able to produce simple words, such as iwi (you) and mama, and he even took his first steps at the CBCC. After his first year participating in HEART at the CBCC, his speech was more audible, and his grip and balance grew stronger, and his teachers hoped that his progress would eventually lead to more advanced educational opportunities in the future.

For students who have more specific needs than Joseph and require more support than the CBCC/Children's Corners can provide, facilitators also collaborate with more specialized community support services and extension workers to ensure that children who need additional services are referred accordingly.

As a component of their comprehensive package of interventions for children, Save the Children in Malawi has noted that HEART for All is a low-cost, scalable model for integrating stimulation, play, creative learning, and psychosocial support for children with disabilities. It can be adapted to almost any context, including emergencies, resource-constrained environments, and areas where adult facilitators have lower educational levels than standard teacher certification. The program has been sustained in Zomba by various community stakeholders, including seasoned HEART facilitators who provide technical mentorship and by Community-Based Organizations and Preschool Networks. Initiatives to provide resources locally and oversight by local implementing partners and government extension workers have also contributed to program stability.

Mexico

Research conducted by Save the Children indicates that only 10% of teachers and education assistants in Early Childhood Care and Development (ECCD) centers in Mexico have been trained to work with children with disabilities, even though children with disabilities are enrolled in their programs. In 2019, building on four years of experience implementing HEART in shelters, schools, preschools, and community centers, Save the Children began piloting HEART for All. To date, the team has rolled out HEART for All in 136 ECCD centers in Mexico City and Estado de México.

Facilitators implementing HEART for All in ECCD centers described the gradual process through which children began to engage with the activities in their own time. One child, Maria, who experienced difficulties communicating and socializing with her peers, reportedly did not want to participate at first, and her teacher found it difficult to keep her interested in the activities. Over time, her teacher began noticing Maria's preferences for different types of materials—for example, working with sponges instead of paintbrushes. Maria's teacher used her observations to make adaptations and provide options for Maria to engage with the materials she felt more comfortable with. "Little by little, she got used to it," so much so that by the end of the school year, she regularly expressed herself both through her artwork and through participating in sharing circles. Throughout the school year, her teacher reported observing her slowly gain greater control over her body (both fine and gross motor skills) and becoming more focused and attentive during various classroom activities. As her communication improved, she became more integrated in the group and

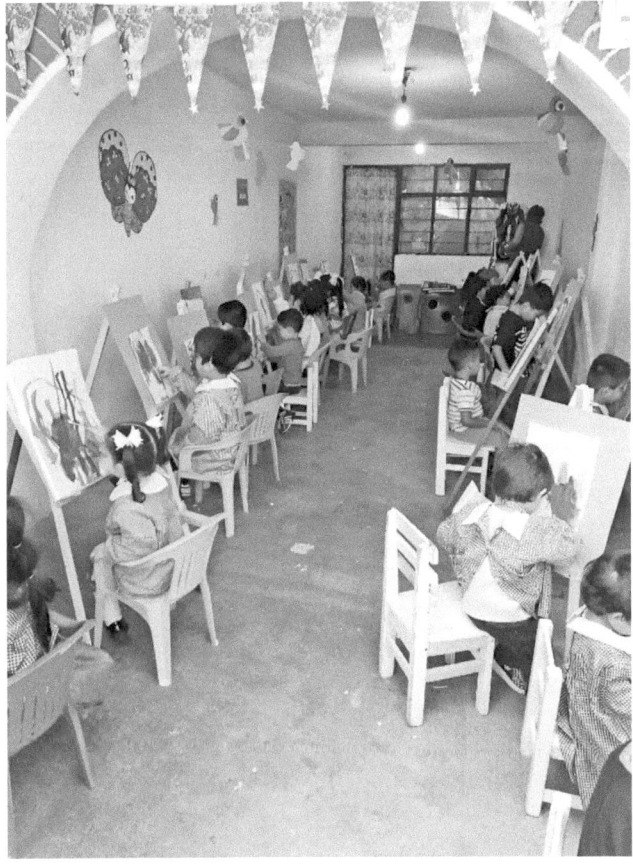

Figure 7.5 Children participate in HEART at a preschool in Mexico

Source: Save the Children

required less direct support from her teacher to participate in HEART activities and other activities in the preschool.

Teachers at other preschools in Mexico have reported finding HEART to be useful for children with disabilities. One preschool attended by several children with developmental delays found that the children's language skills improved as they became more independent and capable of making themselves understood through the HEART sessions. Teachers also reported that they found painting and music activities to be especially effective for children with development delays, helping them to relax, be patient with their creative process, and better able to communicate with other children, including children without development delays, bringing more "tranquility" to the classroom.

Teachers in Mexico also noted that providing different options for materials and different physical arrangements in the classroom were particularly useful for including children with disabilities in the HEART sessions. For example, during painting or drawing activities, children could sit on the floor and paint on paper on the floor in front of them, sit on a chair and paint on paper on a desk or table, or sit or stand and paint on paper attached to the wall or held on an easel. Providing multiple physical space options at one time, along with multiple options for materials, allows both children with and without disabilities to participate in the same activity in the same space at the same time, each engaging in the way that works best for them.

Discussion

Ensuring that psychosocial support programs are fully accessible and adaptable for children with disabilities creates a program and an environment that benefits all children. By providing intentionally accessible and varied options for participating in HEART activities, children are afforded more flexibility and choice to engage with activities in the way that works best for them. Whereas this concept has been long-established in education under the framework of Universal Design for Learning, it is newer to PSS programs, which are often not inclusive of children with disabilities.

Conclusion

HEART for All, while still implemented on a smaller scale than the broader HEART program, has now reached thousands of children with disabilities across multiple countries. The feedback on this program has been overwhelmingly positive, with children, facilitators, and parents experiencing positive growth and development through participation in the program. While adults practice new approaches for engaging with and supporting children with disabilities, the children themselves are given an opportunity to communicate and collaborate with their peers and to develop key social and educational milestones. At the same time, no one intervention is a comprehensive solution for the challenges and barriers faced by children with disabilities and their families. Children need to engage at their own rate of comfort, which may include beginning by simply observing the activities. It takes time for children to be ready to participate, and some children with more severe disabilities may initially find it easier to engage in free art rather than structured art activities. Ultimately, teachers need to remain adaptive and flexible and to celebrate individual successes and accomplishments as they come up. As with any program, the approach and style of the individual facilitator influence how activities are delivered. Because flexibility, patience, and personal commitment to meaningfully including children with disabilities are foundational qualities required for HEART for All to be implemented effectively, a lesson learned is that the selection of adult facilitators is as important as the training that they will receive. In the previously described examples, fortunately the facilitators already had a personal interest and commitment to disability inclusion, and those in Georgia and Albania already had extensive experience working with children with disabilities. As HEART for All continues to expand, it will be important to monitor, document, and promote the necessary prerequisites for facilitators to be able to effectively deliver the program to children. Furthermore, because all children are unique, and some require more complex support than others, education, health, and social programs for children with disabilities should plan to adapt or link to multiple supplemental programs in addition to HEART or other arts-based or psychosocial-focused interventions. This step can best be done through increased multisectoral coordination and collaboration in both global development and humanitarian response programming across the globe.

Key Takeaways

- HEART for All offers an inclusive programming option for children with disabilities, a group often left behind by traditional psychosocial support programs.
- Participation in HEART for All has been linked to skill development as well as to positive cognitive and social outcomes.
- HEART for All works best when facilitators are flexible and adaptive, identifying the individual needs and preferences of their students and making adjustments to better accommodate children with disabilities.
- HEART for All provides all children, including children with disabilities, with an opportunity to be included and engaged, fostering a sense of belonging and overall improved psychosocial well-being.
- HEART for All presents an opportunity for children with disabilities, their caregivers, and their teachers to communicate more openly and build deeper

relationships, which can also transform the adults' own perceptions of inclusion.

Note

1 Behavior is subjective and expectations of children's behavior vary from one context to another. HEART helps teachers and other child support facilitators gain an understanding of children's behavior and shift from an approach of "right and wrong" behavior to one of increased understanding and supportive response. Teacher/facilitator reflections on changes in children's "behavior" during HEART often parallels a change in their own perception of how children should "behave" in different settings, conditions, and contexts.

Chapter 8

HEART for Parents and Caregivers

May Aoun, Rebekka Dieterich-Hartwell, and Laila Sabbagh

The Arts as a Promoter of Parent and Caregiver Well-Being

Parent and Caregiver Well-Being and Parenting

We know how to raise our children, we definitely know what we should or should not do, we understand that yelling, shouting or corporal punishment might be harmful, but with all the stress we are facing, with the level of challenges, it is out of our control, and we end up acting out on our children. We just need a space to vent.

(Refugee Parent in Lebanon)

This desperate appeal of a Syrian refugee parent in Lebanon is indicative of the emotional state numerous parents and caregivers (PCGs) find themselves in as they wrestle with adversities in their lives and crave support to decrease their stress levels. The field experiences from Save the Children programs around the world have shown that the well-being of PCGs has a direct impact on children's well-being and on their physical, cognitive, and psychological development (CDC, 2022). Research confirms that PCGs who struggle with mental health issues and psychosocial well-being are significantly less likely to engage in interactive and positive parenting practices such as nurturing, stimulating, and playing with their child (WHO, 2008). Dealing with these issues is a particular challenge for PCGs in humanitarian and vulnerable settings in which individuals are frequently exposed to extreme stressors, including conflicts, disease outbreaks, natural disasters, poverty, war, and violence, all of which negatively impact their well-being and put strains on relationships (WHO, 2020). In contrast, PCGs who are provided with supported to cope with life's stressors and can build a strong parent–child relationship can promote a child's resilience and protect against early childhood risk factors (Ling, Zahry, & Liu, 2021). One

DOI: 10.4324/9781003367529-9

valuable form of stress management is engagement with the expressive arts, including visual art, music, drama, and dance (Fancourt & Finn, 2019).

Expressive Arts for Parenting and Well-Being

Several research studies have shown that engagement with the expressive arts can be beneficial for PCGs. A recent phenomenological study by Aithal Karkou, and Kuppusamy (2020) found that a dance/movement therapy intervention for parents of children on the autism spectrum increased their resilience and well-being and reduced their stress levels. In a similar setting and using both qualitative and quantitative measures, Champagne and MacDonald (2022) found that dance/movement therapy was perceived as self-expanding and burden-relieving by parents of children on the autism spectrum. Music activities, too, were found to have positive effects on parents of children with autism because they promoted a decrease in stress and improved the parents' quality of life (Gottfried, Elefant, & Gold, 2022). Art therapy for parents of children with chronic pain was found to produce an increased sense of support and validation among participants (Pielech, Sieberg, & Simons, 2013). Engagement with art, movement, or music, particularly in a group setting, thus appears to provide a valuable method of support for PCGs who are dealing with demanding situations at home.

Another area of benefit regarding expressive arts and families is the fostering of improved relationships between PCGs and their children. Expressive arts for children and their caregivers can enhance communication and positive relationships within families (Hoshino & Cameron, 2008). Thompson (2012) found that music activities facilitated by a music therapist in the home environment led to increased interpersonal engagement between children on the autism spectrum and their caregivers through emotional synchronicity, attunement, and provision of structure. Working with toddlers and their parents in Canada, art therapist Proulx (2002) noted that the medium could foster emotionally safe spaces for children and parents to interact and could ultimately encourage the growth of the parent–child relationship. Creative arts engagement programs for caregivers and their children have demonstrated improved child–caregiver relationships as well as increased school attendance and literacy outcomes (Vaughan & Caldwell, 2017).

These clinical examples demonstrate how expressive arts can be effective in fostering positive relationships between PCGs and their children and can increase well-being for families. Although many of these studies are based in North America, HEART has made efforts internationally and in vulnerable settings to include parents and families in art-based psychosocial support programs. We next turn to specific examples of non-clinical expressive arts programming from HEART for parents and caregivers in Bosnia Herzegovina, Mexico, Syria, and Lebanon.

Art Approaches in Practice: HEART for Parents and Caregivers

The HEART program was initially developed as a program to enhance children's psychosocial well-being in vulnerable settings. Over time, through various interactions with PCGs, such as "Community HEART Days" where the entire community is invited to the school or center to experience a special HEART activity together, the benefit of HEART for adults and the interest of PCGs in participating increased. As a result, several different activities emerged in different countries, including after-school programming for children and PCGs to participate in HEART together in Bosnia Herzegovina. HEART-adapted sessions for parents and caregivers organized weekly in Syria and biweekly in Mexico, focused on the psychosocial well-being of the parents and caregivers themselves. These three local country-specific examples influenced the eventual standardization of a global HEART adaptation for parents and caregivers.

The PCGs that participated, together with their children, in a special two-month, after-school HEART program in Bosnia Herzegovina reported a direct positive impact on their own well-being, including feeling calm after relaxation exercises, a stronger sense of connection with others through the sharing-circle process, and an improvement in their parenting skills as illustrated by the following example.

Too Old to Play

In Bosnia Herzegovina, Save the Children initially did not have any HEART experiences with parents and caregivers. The program was planned only for children. Following their first few weeks of HEART sessions, children started talking about the program outside of their schools and community centers. The adults (mainly parents and caregivers) became interested in what HEART was and what their children were doing, so the local HEART team organized a two-month after-school HEART program through which PCGs were invited to attend HEART twice a week with their children. The HEART facilitators discovered that most of the PCGs were already familiar with some of the relaxation activities, such as "Flower and Candle" (when, through dramatic play, the group pretends to smell a flower and blow out a candle to facilitate focused breathing) because the children demonstrated them at home. Most of the participating PCGs reported that they considered themselves too old to play and had forgotten how important it was to engage in fun activities with their children and that, after their participation in HEART, they felt more motivated to play with their children and felt more attached to them through this creative process that helped them communicate in new ways.

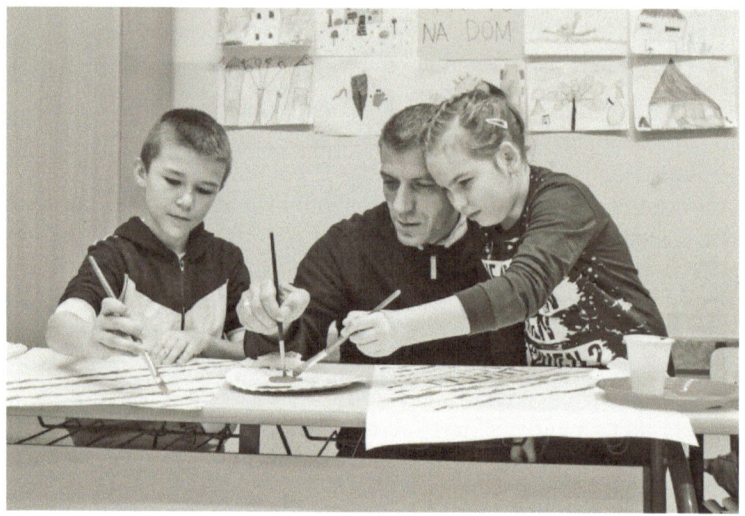

Figure 8.1 Children participate in HEART with their father in Bosnia and Herzegovina

Source: Save the Children

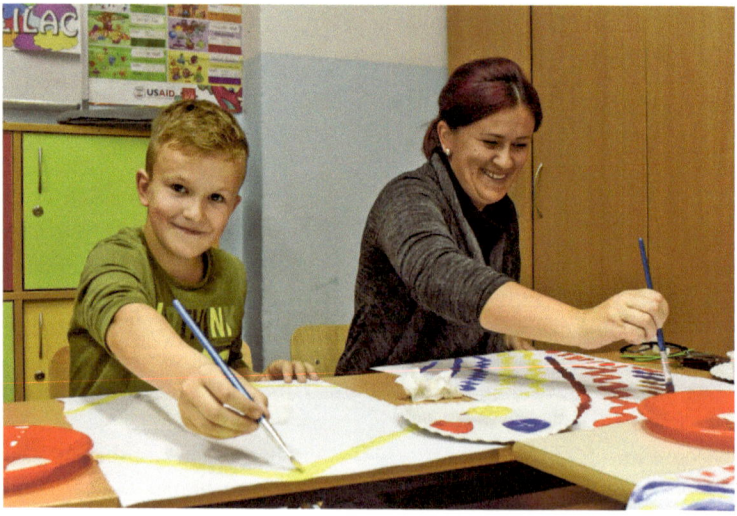

Figure 8.2 A child and his mother participate in HEART in Bosnia and Herzegovina

Source: Save the Children

HEART for the Well-Being of Parents and Caregivers

The psychosocial well-being of parents and caregivers is inextricably linked to their caregiving skills and their children's well-being. An emerging body of research indicates that active arts engagement can enhance adult health and well-being (Fancourt & Finn, 2019). In many contexts of adversity, parents and caregivers struggle to cope with stress and want access to psychosocial support. However, in many settings, field experiences have demonstrated that opportunities for parents and caregivers or other adults to engage in creative and expressive arts activities, or other psychosocial support approaches, are not widely available. Indeed, most existing interventions targeting PCGs in these settings promote positive parenting and the reduction of harsh discipline practices, focusing on improving how parents support children, without addressing the psychological well-being of the caregivers themselves (Pederson et al., 2019). The global success of HEART's art-based psychosocial support program with children and youth in addition to the positive results experienced when demonstrated with PCGs prompted some contexts to use the program specifically for PCG well-being.

Another example of the local utilization of HEART to support PCG well-being, before a standardized adaptation of HEART for adults was developed, is described below.

Caregivers Need Art Too!

Following her first participation in a HEART training session, which was designed to strengthen local staff capacity to support the expansion of HEART programming for children in Syria, a Save the Children staff member, working closely with communities in Northeast Syria, insisted on facilitating the HEART program with a group of lactating and breast-feeding women enrolled in a local nutrition program. Despite skepticism from some of her colleagues, who were not convinced that a children's program based on arts would be accepted by adults in conservative communities, she developed a plan based on the participants' needs and started offering HEART sessions to the mothers in the nutrition group once per week for a three-month period. The results were extremely encouraging. All the women who participated shared that they enjoyed the engagement with art immensely. In addition, they reported using HEART relaxation activities in their daily lives whenever they felt overwhelmed. They also expressed a desire for further sessions, continuing the opportunity for these mothers to support each other through arts and supportive dialogue.

Evidence from Mexico

Children, families, and communities in many parts of Mexico experience adversities that can cause chronic or recurrent stress. Social inequities, poverty, and other stressful situations such as instability, violence, lack of safety, and financial and family problems, are some of the leading causes for frequent emotional distress and mental health problems among vulnerable communities in Mexico (Berenzon et al., 2009). Natural disasters, poverty, and violence cause stress for everyone in the community. Thus, strategies designed to provide psychosocial support need to focus on the children, their parents and other caregivers, and the broader community.

In Mexico City, Save the Children's HEART programming has focused on the geographical districts most heavily affected by poverty and community-based violence. The HEART program has been locally adapted and implemented to support parents and other caregivers—mainly mothers, a few fathers, and other primary and secondary caregivers including grandmothers, uncles, and aunts—of children attending preschools with HEART. In some locations, PCG HEART sessions are conducted in parallel with children's HEART sessions or other child-support activities during the school day at the preschools. In other locations, the PCG HEART sessions are organized after school or on weekends (to accommodate PCG work schedules). In the first year of PCG HEART programming in Mexico, each group of PCGs received 90-minute HEART sessions twice per week for a period of two months per group. Each session included relaxation activities and an expressive art-making activity followed by a sharing circle. The facilitators were mostly preschool teachers trained to facilitate HEART with children and a few Save the Children HEART staff members who supported the teachers for the first few cycles (support included co-facilitating sessions and providing extra arts materials to the preschool when needed).

To assess the impact of HEART programming at preschools in Mexico City, an evaluation was planned at the end of the school year in 2019. The goal of the evaluation was to understand the impact that HEART had on children, PCGs, and teachers. Interviews were conducted with PCGs, focusing on changes that they observed in their children and in themselves, as well as any strengths and challenges experienced while participating in the program. Most commonly, PCGs responded that HEART taught them how to better manage their stress and improve their emotional expression. They gave examples of using deep breathing, meditation, taking more time to calm down, rationalizing their emotions, and listening to music to relax. For example, one mother stated, "Almost all the time I'm stressed … I get home and then what I do is I sit down, I play relaxing music, and I do all the exercises that we were taught here. In the end I feel calmer. I feel more relaxed in my neck and calmer internally and externally." In addition, parents often reported that this experience deepened their parent–child relationship. as One mother shared "It is about being able to integrate into an activity together, recognize each other, feel, listen, speak, that is the basis of the program." Many PCGs reported that their experience with HEART helped them feel closer to their children and to be more attuned to their children's needs. PCGs shared examples of how the program helped them to better understand what their children needed from them and the importance of being patient, empathetic, and compassionate with their children. PCGs also noted that they continued to use HEART activities at home with their children even after the program for parents and caregivers ended and that this was easy to do because they were provided a bag of arts supplies to take home (provided by Save the Children and the preschool) (Pisani et al., 2021).

In addition to being asked about their own experiences, the PCGs were asked about what changes they observed in their children, because their children also participated in HEART over the course of a full school year. The positive reflections provided by the PCGs on the program's impact on their children[1] complemented their own experiences and highlighted how supporting both children and their PCGs created a continuum of support between the school and the home (Pisani et al., 2021).

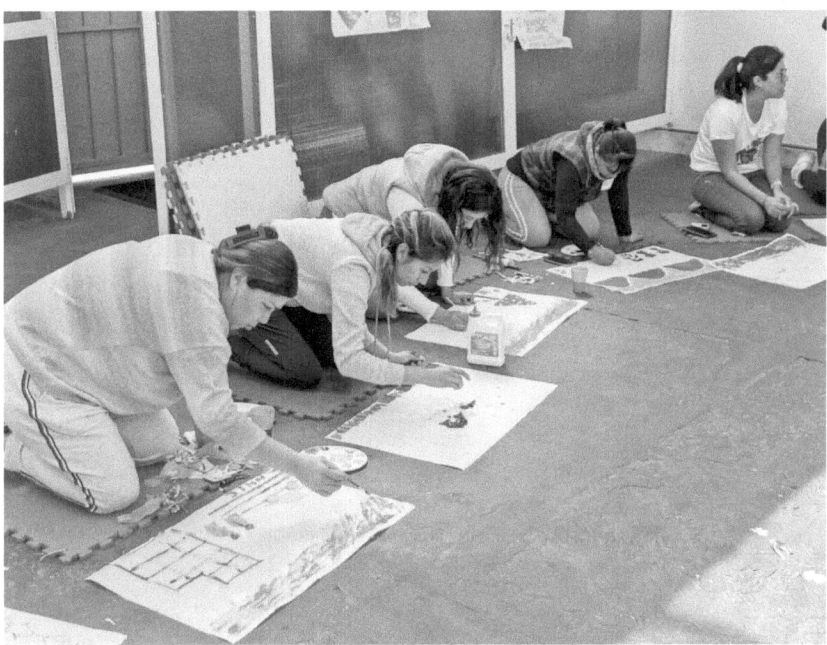

Figure 8.3 Mothers participate in HEART in Mexico
Source: Save the Children

The following example demonstrates how one mother experienced changes in her relationship with her son over the course of her participation in HEART in parallel to his participation.

In My Son's Shoes

My son [and I are both] participating in the HEART program. I really like the program … it is a wonderful tool. [It has been] a very good experience and has helped me to put myself in my son's shoes on many occasions. Sometimes adult life absorbs you and you forget that you were a child once. The program makes me understand children more and provides the opportunity to play more with my son and get everything out and rethink my life from my roots. HEART has helped me to be more patient with my son. Before, I used to get very angry; now I see him with different eyes. I am more grounded. I let him express his emotions, his sadness and anger because I learned that it is useless for me to get angry with him and him get angry with me.

The Parent and Caregiver Peer Support Group Program

The success of the HEART adaptations for parents and caregivers that were done in several countries, coupled with the high demand for mental health and psychosocial support programs following the COVID-19 pandemic in 2020, led to the development of the Parent and Caregiver Peer Support Group Program, the standardized global adaptation of HEART for PCGs. The main objective of this intervention is to support stress processing through creative self-expression, enhance supportive social connections, and promote self-care among the parents and caregivers of children attending Save the Children-supported programming. It is an important step in HEART's promotion of a socioecological model that provides arts-based psychosocial support for children, PCGs, and communities affected by adversity.

The program is intentionally designed to address specific challenges that Save the Children has encountered with MHPSS programming globally. The first challenge is related to the stigma of mental health programming. Programs that are labeled as "mental health" or "MHPSS" are sometimes not accepted due to stigma around mental health, especially when provided in clinical mental health settings such as hospitals or health clinics. The peer support groups are intentionally facilitated by non-mental health professionals such as paraprofessional social workers, teachers, or other community support staff. The name and design of the program (peer support and expressive arts), along with the non-specialized facilitation, contribute to the program being accepted in a range of communities that might otherwise reject MHPSS programs. The second challenge relates to parenting programs, which often focus on the parenting skills of adult facilitators rather than on the well-being of the caregivers themselves. During the program pilots in Lebanon and Syria, participants regularly provided positive feedback about how much they appreciated a program that supported them directly and did not lecture them about how to be better parents. Although the program demonstrates positive ways of supporting self-expression and stress processing, it does so without specific messaging on negative parenting methods but rather allows caregivers to experience psychosocial support for themselves, which in turn strengthens their abilities to provide similar support to their children. The third challenge is related to literacy. Because the program does not require participants to read or write but provides verbal guidance and facilitation with artistic expression, it is available to support parents and caregivers with varying levels of literacy.

This adaptation of HEART for parents and caregivers consists of weekly or biweekly structured sessions of 90 minutes each, in groups of 8 to 15 participants. Each structured session includes mindfulness and relaxation activities, expressive drawing on a specific topic or theme, a sharing and support circle, a grounding activity, and a self-care reflection, as well as self-care homework. Additionally, chat and connect sessions can be added regularly or on an ad-hoc basis. The chat and connect sessions are mainly open discussion opportunities where no specific theme is discussed, but participants and facilitators simply share anything on their minds, and the discussion flows as needed. These open discussion sessions can start with a short relaxation activity and end with a grounding activity or a self-care reflection/commitment and can be as short as 30 minutes or as long as a standard 90-minute session.

The goal of the program is to provide long-term psychosocial support in multiple phases. The program can run over an extended period, starting with eight structured sessions in its first phase. Depending on the context and needs of the participants, the program can be extended to a second and a third phase should parents and caregivers choose to continue with their groups. In the last two phases, participants decide the frequency, regularity, and duration of sessions and whether they are structured or chat and connect sessions or a mixture of both. The PCG sessions are led by two facilitators. All facilitators attend a three-day training program, complemented with a refresher training session after three months of implementation. In addition, facilitators attend regular group supervision sessions with an experienced mental health supervisor. Facilitators are most often community support workers such as community social workers or community health workers or school-based support staff such as teachers or school counselors. In some settings, the facilitators are unique to the PCG support program and in other settings they facilitate both HEART with children and the Parent Caregiver Peer Support Group with PCGs.

To support a simple, low-cost model that can be used in various contexts, often added onto an existing HEART program for children, or integrated into a community support space that might not have storage available, the PCG support program uses basic arts supplies, most often including paper and crayons (or other writing and drawing utensils).[2] Additional arts materials can be added if locally available and cost effective and if time and space allow for more diverse art modalities to be used. Within the design of the program, each local context has the flexibility to add additional expressive arts activities or local and traditional arts, as appropriate.

The first two countries to pilot this standardized global adaptation of HEART for adults were Lebanon and Syria. Below, we offer some insights and examples from these first two pilots of the program. It is important to note that in both countries, the Parent and Caregiver Peer Support Group Program is not a stand-alone program but is rather part of a comprehensive MHPSS approach whose goal is to enhance psychosocial well-being and strengthen the local protective environment for children and their families.

The Local Context in Syria

For more than 12 years, Syria has experienced a complex humanitarian emergency. The ongoing conflict has caused widespread destruction of civilian infrastructure, economic hardship, and the largest number of internally displaced people (IDPs) in the world (The World Bank, 2016), with one in three Syrians experiencing internal displacement in 2022 (UNHCR, The UN Refugee Agency, 2023a). The conflict inevitably has had far-reaching and lasting consequences on the mental health and psychosocial well-being of children, families, and communities. Northeast Syria is highly impacted by the armed conflict and by the displacement problem, with more than 700,000 IDPs who are almost entirely dependent on humanitarian assistance. One of the most challenging settings in Northeast Syria is an IDP camp that hosts over 60,000 people, mostly Syrian and Iraqi women and children, as well as women and children from 60 other countries across the world who are often referred to as third country nationals (TCNs) (Save the Children, 2021d). Because of the diverse and sensitive contexts from which many of the women and children in the camp originate, many misconceptions exist based on stereotypes and lack of understanding about the countries, conflicts, and cultures from which the women and children originate. These misconceptions often limit communication, interaction, and support among the women and their families and between them and the support workers in the camp. Because the camp's residents have a diverse background with complex personal histories and significant psychosocial support needs, it is important to create emotionally safe and supportive spaces for communication and bonding among children, caregivers, and staff, to break down barriers and foster a supportive community for everyone in the camp.

Save the Children supports diverse multi-sectoral services in the camp, including education, protection, nutrition, health, and hygiene programming. MHPSS is integrated into several of these sectors and the first pilot of the Parent and Caregiver Peer Support Group Program launched in February 2023 in community centers, supporting approximately 100 female parents and caregivers aged 25–55 years old. The support groups ran twice a week, including one Structured Session and one Chat & Connect Session. The two case stories below showcase the positive impact of the program during this first pilot.

Unveiling My True Self (Save the Children Facilitator, Northeast Syria)

The "Mask" activity resulted in profound participation, even though we as facilitators were concerned that this activity would not be culturally accepted. To our surprise, in the camp, there was intense sharing happening among participants. One mother confided that she was very scared of us facilitators. *"We knew that you were afraid of us as well. We also knew that you had misconceptions about us. The activities we did together, and the mask activity in particular, broke down many barriers so we were able to remove our 'masks' and show you our true faces. This activity allowed us to get closer with you and each other and build trust within the group."* The mother also shared that participants are now comfortable showing their true selves and that they allowed facilitators to *"see their emotions and talk with us, like any mother or wife, that we can laugh, cry and joke; and that we are not just stereotypes."* She added: *"We are at a stage where we shed all our masks and are acting like ourselves again."*

Filling the Void (Mother, Syria)

I was suffering from loneliness and emptiness after my husband traveled to Europe, leaving me alone with two children. … I moved to live with my extended family, but this increased the psychological pressure on me … My loneliness was not due to the lack of people around me, but I was feeling empty from inside … I decided to attend the PCGs sessions to spend some time outside the house. We used to meet in a calm and safe atmosphere, away from the hustle and bustle … Today, after participating in numerous sessions, I feel that I have filled the void in me, and I have decreased my stress and begun to express myself calmly and firmly. Perhaps the most prominent thing that I experienced after the sessions was the change in the way I discipline my children, as I began to move away from harsh discipline in dealing with them to avoid causing them any psychological distress … The relaxation activities I learned became positive reinforcement for the children to behave during the day so we could practice the self-care homework together in the evening ... After these sessions, I became more flexible, calm, and able to control my anger and tend to my stress and the needs of my children.

The Local Context in Lebanon

In recent years, Lebanon experienced an economic collapse, political instability, and the ongoing challenge of hosting one of the largest populations of Syrian refugees in the region for more than a decade. More than one million Syrian civilians have fled the war in Syria and sought refuge in Lebanon. The majority of the Syrian refugees living in Lebanon live in rented accommodations, disused buildings, or informal tent settlements, because there are no formal refugee camps set up in the country.[3] Save the Children's MHPSS work is mostly integrated into education and child protection activities including support for pre-schools, after-school programs, alternative learning programs for out-of-school children, youth programs, community centers for children and families, and parent/caregiver support initiatives.

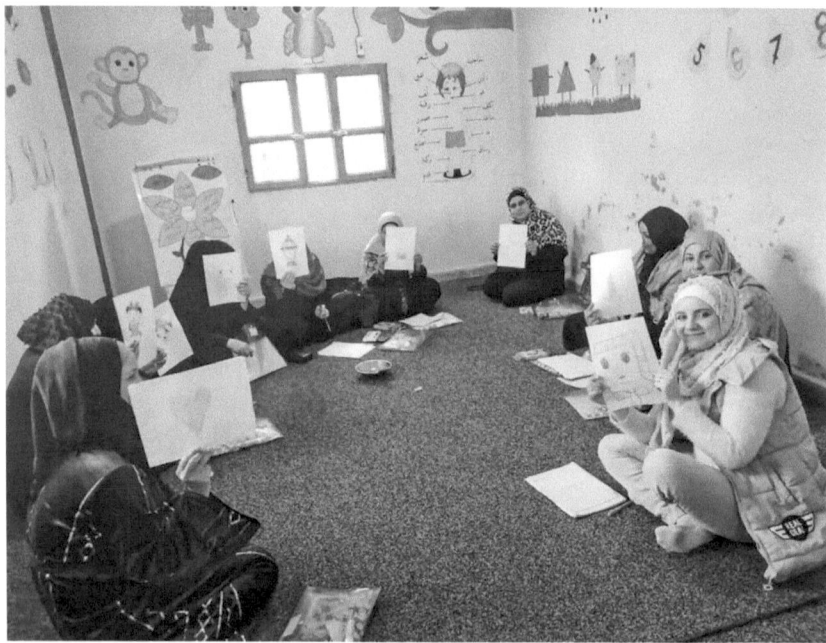

Figure 8.4 Mothers participate in a HEART-adapted peer support group in Syria

Source: Save the Children

HEART has been used to support children in Lebanon since 2016, in pre-schools, after-school programs, and community centers. The Parent and Caregiver Peer Support Group Program was first piloted in Lebanon in 2022. During the pilot, the program was implemented once a week for groups of approximately 10 to15 parents and caregivers, with a total of 350 participants across two regions in Lebanon (Beirut and Beqaa). The majority of PCGs who participated in the program pilot were Syrian refugees along with some Lebanese nationals from the local host community. Most of the groups consisted of mothers and other female caregivers, in addition to two groups of fathers and male caregivers, and one mixed gender group. In most locations, the program was facilitated in community centers except in one location where it was implemented in tents. The following case examples demonstrate the experience of the parents and caregivers during the first program pilot in Lebanon.

Men Also Need Support! (Facilitator, Lebanon)

I was surprised to see how much the men enjoyed the sessions. Not one of them dropped out of the group. They continually told us that they looked forward to the session each time and found them very interesting. They were actually upset if a session was postponed! During the expressive drawing activity, they took their time to draw and color, they talked during the sharing circle, and although they told us that they liked everything we did, they said their favorite part was the relaxation activities. Many of the men told us that these sessions really positively impacted their lives, and that self-care was something they had never thought about before. The sessions gave them the time to do things they enjoy but never had time to do. They also told us that the sessions helped them express and release bottled-up thoughts and emotions, and that this transformed their mood as they were surrounded by people who were also weighed down by similar concerns and worries. The sessions helped them make the time and have the space to talk and de-stress together, which helped them to be more present and more positive in their relationships with their families.

Tears Connect Us (Female Facilitator, Lebanon)

During a session following the earthquake (in Turkey and Syria), there was a lot of fear and anxiety that more aftershocks would follow. I felt that I should be helping and be useful and was feeling powerless where I was (in Lebanon). While facilitating the group session, the activity "what makes you feel hopeful" triggered me. I started crying as I could not find a reason for hope at that moment. I left the session and handed it over to my co-facilitator, but when I returned, I discovered that all the participants were crying. I felt guilty as I was the reason for all the tears; instead of lowering participants' stress, I felt that I had increased it exponentially. I sat down with the participants in the circle, and they began sharing spontaneously about their worries and fears. I ended the discussion with a grounding activity. During the following session, the participants said that our crying circle was a major relief for them and that they felt close to me for having cried and for sharing my emotions. Also, the fact that they cried and let out their emotions helped them put words to their pain, express themselves, and return home with less anxiety. It is important that we have the space to share these feelings and to support each other, because we are all dealing with so much. As a facilitator, this group helped me, because I wasn't just there to facilitate the process for them, but I was part of it too, we were all doing it together. This group helped many of us to find supportive community we didn't have before, or didn't prioritize before, and now we do."

Evidence from Program Pilots in Lebanon and Syria

Thank you for these sessions, no one thought about us before, thank you for providing us with the space to just be as adults, as human beings, and not just as caregivers.

(A mother in Lebanon)

Following the implementation of the first phase of the Parent and Caregiver Peer Support Group Program, a satisfaction survey was completed by 348 participants in Lebanon and 51 participants in Syria, paired with either key informant interviews or discussions in focus groups composed of participants and facilitators. The questions surveyed the level of participant satisfaction with the program, collected feedback on program logistics and content such as the scheduling and duration of sessions along with activity and discussion topics, and collected participant reflections on how the program impacted their well-being.

Three specific questions related to the program's impact on the subjective well-being of participants were asked, including the impact that participation in the program had on mood, self-care routines, and feelings of social connectedness. In the survey, responses to these three areas were collected using a 5-point Likert scale that allowed for responses including very positive, positive, neutral, negative, or very negative. As seen in the charts below, the survey results demonstrated mostly positive or very positive outcomes on all three indicators in both countries. These results were further supported by participant reflections captured during Key Informant Interviews and Focus Group Discussions.

Positive Impact on Mood in Lebanon and Syria

In Lebanon, 68% of the participants reported that their participation in the peer support groups resulted in a very positive and 31% reported a positive, impact

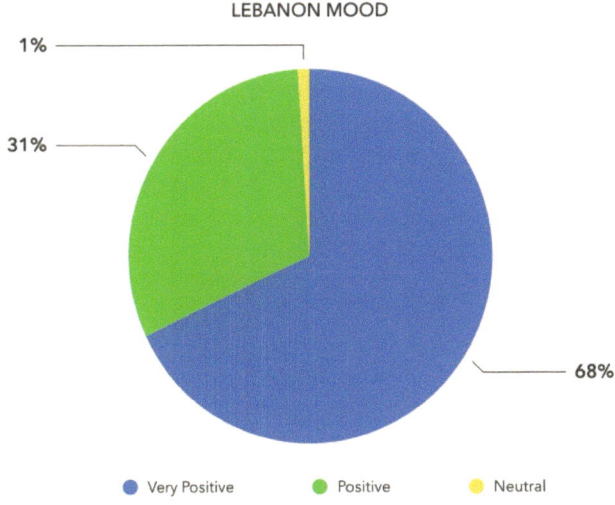

Figure 8.5 Impact on mood in Lebanon

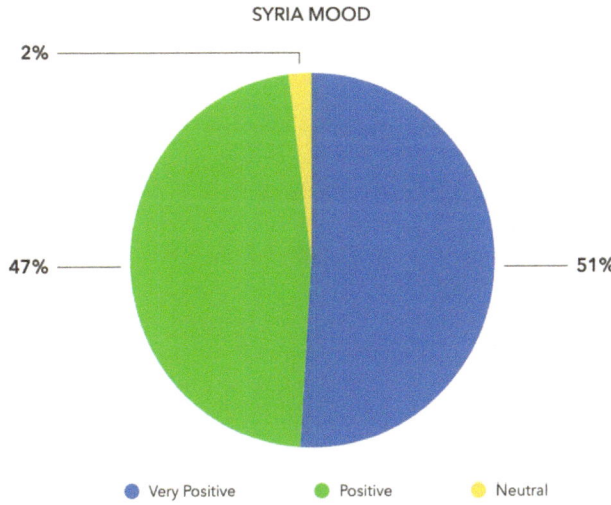

Figure 8.6 Impact on mood in Syria

on their mood, while 1% of respondents in Lebanon had a neutral response (no impact, either positive or negative). In Syria, 51% of respondents reported a very positive impact on mood, with 47% reporting a positive impact and 2% a neutral impact. These overwhelmingly positive results were further supported by reflections during interviews and focus group discussions that revealed participant perceptions of improved self-worth after completing the first phase of the program. In Lebanon, a participant shared that the program helped her to "realize how valuable I am as a human being and start loving myself." Another mother in Lebanon shared that participating in the program "increased my love toward life since I am now able to dedicate some time for myself." Multiple participants also revealed a sense of being better able to manage stress, which led to improved moods (Save the Children, 2023c). Improved mood is directly related to the other two well-being indicators surveyed: Improved social connections and improved self-care routine can both have positive implications for mood.

Positive Impact on Social Connections in Lebanon and Syria

In Lebanon, 59% of those surveyed reported a very positive and 37% reported a positive impact on social connectedness, with 4% neutral. In Syria, 45% of respondents reported a very positive impact on social connectedness, 51% reported a positive impact, and 4% provided a neutral response. Reflections from interviews and focus group discussions revealed examples of the impact of improved social connectedness experienced through participation in the support groups. In Syria, participants highlighted that they made new friends or strengthened existing relationships with other members of the community. One participant from Syria shared that before the group started, she felt "disconnected from the world" and other participants noted how the new connections they made in the group extended beyond the organized sessions and were now part of everyday life. A mother in Syria shared that she "knew the other participants only superficially before starting the support group; however, after some time, they became close friends" and that during the art-making part of one of the support group sessions, she "sculpted a teapot to express that I was not able to have tea that morning because I was out of gas, so a new friend in the group prepared a pot of tea and offered it to me and my family later that day. This made me very happy and showed how close we are now and how much we support each other" (Save the Children, 2023c).

Another important aspect of the improved social connections is how people from different backgrounds and groups were able to communicate and bond for the first time. In Lebanon, some of the groups included both Syrian refugees and local Lebanese citizens. For many, the groups offered an opportunity to get to know people they otherwise never would have met. In Syria, some of the groups

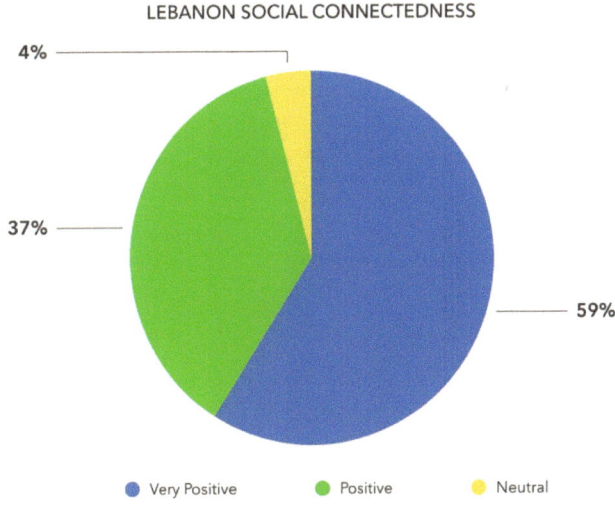

Figure 8.7 Impact on social connectedness in Lebanon

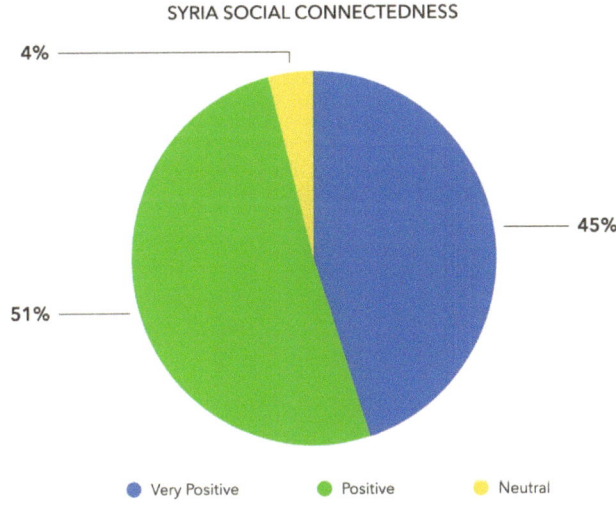

Figure 8.8 Impact on social connectedness in Syria

included non-Syrians (refugees from other countries) who did not speak Arabic. They were able to communicate through the art-making activities (drawing and sculpting) and through miming or acting out things they wanted to share, in addition to the facilitators occasionally using a translation app to assist in communication. The improved social connections strongly linked with self-care routines in that group participants started to spend time together outside of the support group sessions and support each other to practice self-care.

Positive Impact on Self-Care Routines in Lebanon and Syria

The topic of self-care is addressed repeatedly throughout the first phase of the support group program. At the end of each support group session, a homework assignment is given to the participants to practice some type of self-care every day. Reflections on self-care take place regularly with a focus on intentional planning for practical ways to do things every day that promote relaxation and stress processing. In Lebanon, 65% of respondents reported that participating in the program had a very positive impact on their self-care routine, with 32% reporting a positive impact and 3% neutral. In Syria, 45% of participants surveyed reported a very positive, and 53% a positive, impact on self-care routine, with 2% reporting a neutral response. One of the program facilitators in Lebanon noted how surprised she was that the group participants took the

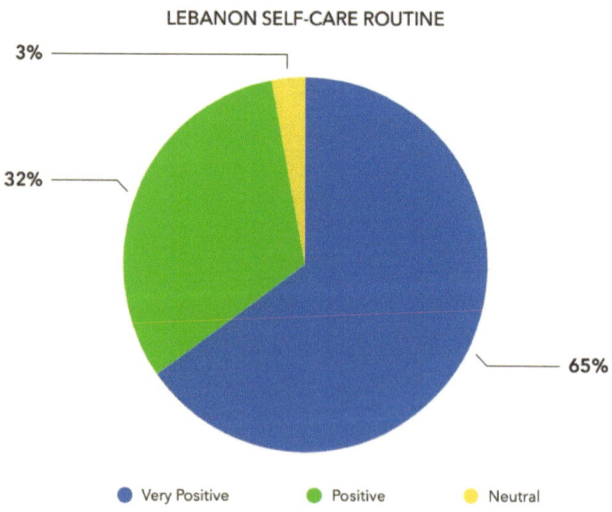

Figure 8.9 Impact on self-care routine in Lebanon

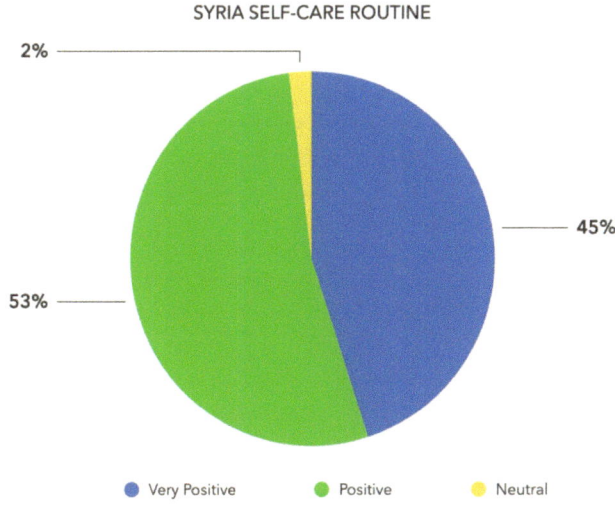

Figure 8.10 Impact on self-care routine in Syria

self-care homework assignment seriously and said, "it is amazing how they are all doing their self-care homework and how they understood how important it is" (Save the Children, 2023c). Many of the facilitators themselves, across multiple countries, struggle with work–life balance and have noted that facilitating the process for others has helped to remind them of the importance of self-care and has improved their own prioritization of it in their everyday lives.

Positive Impact on Home Life

A total of 98% of respondents in Syria and 81% in Lebanon reported that participation in the peer support group had a positive impact on their home life. The local context in each country is important to consider given the very high positive impact reported in Syria where all participants are IDPs and refugees living in formal camps with consistent home environments, whereas in Lebanon the home context is more varied, including both refugees and non-refugees (host community members) living in different home environments.

Examples of positive impacts on home life that were shared during interviews and focus group discussions included impact on the behavior of the parent and on the interaction between the parent and other household members such as children and other adults in the home. Many of the participants reported that they learned to better handle and process stress and negative emotions through the support group. They noted that intentionally taking more time to calm down including using deep breathing exercises and meditation techniques when feeling stressed at home, rationalizing their emotions, and practicing self-care at home helped them to better manage stress.

Many parents shared that the art activities they engaged in during the sessions helped them feel closer to their children because they were expressing themselves in a similar way to their children (through art). They also noted that the process of expressing themselves and paying attention to their own emotions helped them to better understand how their children must feel. They felt that this improved their relationships with their families because they developed more empathy, which improved their ways of communicating with, and nurturing, their children.

Participants also shared that they do many of the arts activities and relaxation activities with their children at home. The PCGs gave examples of how the activities have helped them better understand their young children's needs and to respond to them more effectively and patiently. When asked what she learned from the PCG support group sessions, one mother in Lebanon stated, "to be tolerant, to get closer to my daughter". Another mother in Syria shared, "I used to explode (with anger) faster and take it out on my children, now I feel more calm and I'm happy that I interact better with my daughters". Parents also reported sharing relaxation activities with their spouses, family members, or friends as illustrated by a Lebanese mother, "in the evening, I gather my children and my husband, and we do the relaxation activities together."

Cultural and Social Experiences

The positive relationships built between participants in the support groups led to the integration of cultural and social experiences both within the organized group sessions and beyond. In Syria, during the chat and connect sessions, the women took the opportunity to share holiday recipes they cook for their families and even started cooking and sharing food together (bringing food and tea to the sessions to share during their chats). Also in Syria, the groups sang songs and shared stories about their favorite music, and some of the groups did a henna ritual[4] as a closing activity after the first phase of the support groups ended.

Desire to Continue

In many locations there were requests to continue the program beyond the first stage of the pilot. All surveyed participants reported that they would recommend the groups to others, and multiple participants from Lebanon indicated that they considered the sessions a form of self-care that benefitted their daily life and that they would struggle to maintain their well-being without the organized group. Thus, the flexibility of the program to continue beyond phase 1, with additional phases of both Structured Sessions and Chat and Connect Sessions, and the option to continue as a community group without formal facilitation after phase 3 (to continue with participant-led Chat & Connect sessions) is of particular relevance to providing sustained psychosocial support over an extended time period, particularly in contexts of chronic adversity.

Challenges and Recommendations

One of the most significant challenges of the program implementation was with mothers of infants or toddlers who had to bring the children to the group meetings (children too young to participate in parallel child-support activities that most often focus on children aged 3 to 18). This situation necessitated a safe space and additional staff for the children where they were entertained and supervised so that their mothers could attend the sessions. This learning experience will influence the logistics of future support groups to ensure that the PCG groups have childcare options to support caregiver participation.

Another major challenge was getting fathers to sign up for the program. Overall, the participation of fathers and other male caregivers in the program was low, but those that did participate had a very positive experience, and all reported that they would recommend the program to others. Part of the challenge of male caregiver engagement was with the scheduling of the sessions, which took place during the day when many male caregivers were working and thus not available to attend. One of the recommendations for Syria and Lebanon is thus to adapt the session timing to accommodate the schedules of male caregivers in this context,[5] which requires flexibility in staff scheduling. An important aspect of this type of work is to ensure human resource policies that allow staff to work hours that correspond to programming needs, which often means outside of a typical 9 am–5 pm workday.

Discussion

The lack of programming examples and studies that examine the role of the arts in addressing the needs of parents and caregivers living in conditions of adversity, specifically within the global development and humanitarian sectors, points to a significant gap that programs like HEART can start to fill. The HEART adaptation examples for parents and caregivers demonstrate how expressive arts can be a powerful tool to enhance the well-being of caregivers and, by extension, the well-being of families. The HEART programs' distinct advantages in vulnerable settings include its cost efficiency, adaptability to local contexts, and inclusiveness from gender, disability, and literacy perspectives. Additionally, the fact that these programs can be embedded in community services and facilitated by non-mental-health specialists helps to overcome the frequent stigma associated with mental health interventions. Furthermore, the HEART program also acts to support prevention by addressing mild mental health symptoms through non-specialized support before serious mental health problems occur. Finally, a program for adults that is based on expressive arts and enjoyable experiential activities combined with supportive communication, rather than rigid lecturing and tutoring methods that many parent support programs rely on, provides a new type of emotionally safe and supportive space for parents and caregivers to relax, process stress, and support each other. The approach has demonstrated extremely positive impacts on the mood, social connectedness, and self-care routines of participants and is in demand to be sustained and expanded to reach more parents and caregivers dealing with conditions of adversity. The use of arts-based peer support programming for parents and caregivers is an effective, low-cost, and sustainable model for improving the psychosocial well-being of PCGs within the global development and humanitarian sectors.

Conclusion

Parents and other caregivers who are stressed and do not have a support mechanism to enable them to process and cope with such stress, may perpetuate stress responses at home, limiting their ability to provide a supportive and nurturing environment for their children. This situation worsens the PCG–child relationship and, as a result, increases stress for all family members. It is imperative that PCGs living in conditions of adversity are provided with opportunities to engage in activities to enhance their own well-being, notably expressive art activities. As seen from the experience of the HEART adaptation for adults, expressive arts integrated Parent and Caregiver Peer Support Groups can support the psychosocial well-being of PCGs living in conditions of adversity and enhance their abilities to support the development and well-being of their children.

Key Takeaways

- Parents and caregivers living in conditions of adversity need psychosocial support to improve their own well-being which in turn improves their ability to support the well-being of their children.
- The adaptation of HEART to support parents and caregivers has demonstrated positive impact on the well-being of parents and caregivers in multiple countries and contexts.
- Arts-based psychosocial support is an effective, sustainable, and low-cost approach to supporting the psychosocial well-being of parents and caregivers.

Notes

1 The impact of the HEART program on children in preschool HEART programming in Mexico City, as documented by the 2019 Evaluation in Mexico, is discussed in more detail in Chapter 5.

2   Because the program is more likely (than the HEART program with children) to take place in a community space that does not already have arts supplies or storage space for arts materials available, such as a health clinic or community center, it is important to ensure that the arts supplies needed to facilitate the program are simple, transportable, and not time consuming to set up for each session.

3   Lebanese government policy does not allow for formal refugee camps.

4   The henna ritual used henna paste to draw decorative designs on the hands of the participants (participants decorated each other's hands). It is an activity that is often done to mark the beginning or ending of something important or to celebrate a significant event.

5   The same logistical adaptation would be needed for both male and female caregivers in different settings across the globe. In Mexico and Bosnia Herzegovina, some parent/caregiver support sessions take place during the day and some take place in the evenings, to accommodate the schedules of working caregivers.

Chapter 9

The Role of HEART in Supporting Staff Well-being

Dario Lipovac, Bani Malhotra, and Victoria Schwachter

Introduction

Human beings are attuned to connections with others. Through supportive connections, they can meet needs related to safety, physiology, love, and belonging. Supportive connections are at the core of Save the Children's HEART program and the associated HEART-adapted Peer Support Groups for Adults including both the Parent and Caregiver Peer Support Groups and the Staff Peer Support Groups. Over the years, Save the Children HEART trainers have noted that one of the most consistent comments from participants in post-training feedback is the value of supportive connections and a sense of belonging with their peers that they experience while participating in HEART trainings. Acknowledging the positive response and inspiration that the HEART program and related Adult Peer Support Groups have fostered among participants, this chapter underscores the need for, and the strength of, staff peer support programming within the global humanitarian response and international development sectors.

Global development and humanitarian response work can often be both personally and professionally fulfilling while at the same time stressful. Work environments in contexts of poverty, conflict, displacement, natural disasters, and infectious disease expose staff to chronic and often intense stress. Recurrent and intense exposure to human suffering can lead to a negative impact on psychosocial well-being including negative physical, psychological, and social outcomes for staff. Group-based psychosocial support programming for staff can mitigate such a negative impact and help staff to find supportive social connections that can lead to improved well-being. The experience of the HEART program in supporting staff well-being provides a practical example of how arts-based group psychosocial support can improve staff well-being in different working environments around the world.

DOI: 10.4324/9781003367529-10

Working in International Development and Humanitarian Response

Multiple factors that play a role in staff well-being include unique personal stressors, common local contextual stressors, and specific intense stressors related to working in conditions of adversity or chronic exposure to human suffering, which is common in global development and humanitarian response work. Humanitarian response workers are most often national staff from the local population and affected communities, which means they experience first-hand stress due to living in conditions of adversity and often intensive stress related to their role working to support others in adverse contexts. International humanitarian staff face other stressors linked to working and living in a different culture, away from family and support systems, and often moving from one area of crisis to another. Some humanitarian workers who do not live and work in the affected areas of adversity may still be faced with stressors from remote exposure to stories, images, videos, and other information related to human suffering.

Two key categories of stressors that humanitarian staff experience include operational stressors and organizational stressors. Operational stressors are types of stressors inherent in humanitarian work, such as working long hours, being exposed to adversities in the local setting, and working and living in a stressful environment. Organizational stressors are stressors related to the working environment within a specific organization. Such stressors can include excessive workloads for individuals or teams, lack of support from management, or a workplace culture that discriminates against specific groups of employees (Jachens, 2019). Organizational stressors can lead to negative physical and mental health outcomes including burnout, anxiety, exhaustion, insomnia, and others (CHS Alliance, 2021). Although operational stressors are inherent in humanitarian work, in contrast, organizational stressors can be addressed to mitigate their impact on staff well-being. This chapter focuses on arts-based psychosocial support programming to address *operational stressors* in global development and humanitarian work. However, *organizational stressors* should not be neglected in future publications and/or research on staff well-being.

The Importance of Organizational Support Mechanisms for Staff

Staff working in contexts of adversity are at risk of experiencing negative consequences to their mental and physical health (Ager et al. 2012; Bell, Shanti, & Dalton, 2003; Lopes-Cardozo et al., 2012; Knight, 2013; Mackereth et al., 2005; Maslach, Jackson, & Leiter, 1996). Quality staff well-being approaches can have a positive impact on staff well-being and in turn on work productivity (Chemali et al., 2017). With appropriate support, staff can manage stress and avoid some of the negative consequences associated with working in contexts of adversity by engaging in problem- and emotion-focused strategies (Lazarus and Folkman, 1985). When organizations provide staff well-being support through which humanitarian workers can develop or utilize problem- and emotion-focused strategies that help them cope with operational stressors in parallel to wider support mechanisms that address organizational stressors, a comprehensive, compassionate, and multilayered approach to support staff well-being can mitigate the negative impact of working in conditions of adversity.

The adaptation of HEART to support adults, both parents and staff, includes the use of expressive arts and play to provide group-based psychosocial support to individuals who, to date, range in age from 20 to 75. The benefits of play for adults are significantly less researched than the benefits of play for children (Magnuson and Barnett, 2013) but we know that play can produce positive emotions across multiple age groups and that increased playfulness is associated with higher levels of well-being for all ages (Proyer, 2014). A range of activities that include expressive arts has demonstrated improved social connections, emotional awareness, and well-being among humanitarian staff (Bardot, 2018; Gavron et al., 2022; Kalmanowitz, 2016; Ma & Penner, 2018). Arts and play help mitigate the effects of stress on the brain and can support self-expression and group communication in ways that can improve well-being for both children and adults.

The HEART-adapted Staff Peer Support Group Program highlights the importance of staff taking time to pause, slow down, reflect, and recharge, especially when they are faced with multiple layers of stress related to working in conditions of adversity or working in contexts in which they are regularly exposed (directly or indirectly) to human suffering. HEART-adapted Staff Peer Support Groups have generated positive responses from teachers, community health workers, and Save the Children and partner non-governmental organization (NGO) employees in several countries.

HEART Adaptation: Staff Peer Support Groups

For years, trained HEART facilitators have routinely reported positive changes in their own psychosocial well-being during and after participating in HEART training and while facilitating the program with children and families. Anecdotal reports of this experience have grown alongside the accumulation of evidence about the program's positive impact on children's psychosocial well-being globally.

Impact evaluation of HEART programming in Mexico City's community-based preschools demonstrated positive changes for teachers who participated in HEART training received HEART mentoring from Save the Children HEART trainers, and facilitated the program with children and parents. Teachers reported personal improved self-expression, increased patience and empathy with children, and better personal stress management (Kaimal et al., 2022). The findings from Mexico align with monitoring feedback from HEART facilitators in multiple countries who consistently report that participation in HEART generates a positive impact on their personal well-being and professional lives. Reported benefits include better self-expression and stress management, improved understanding of group bonding and support, more social connectedness with peers, and a perspective shift regarding the importance of expressive arts and play for psychosocial support (for both children and adults).

Inspired by this evidence and feedback, Save the Children developed the Staff Peer Support Group Program (an adaptation of HEART for adults) in 2020 to support the psychosocial well-being of staff involved in different types of work supporting children and families in different contexts of adversity. The first pilot of the program took place during the COVID-19 lockdown, through which approximately 40 staff members in the United States participated in remote video facilitation of the program.[1] It later piloted the program with health workers, Save the Children staff, and NGO partners in Indonesia in 2021, and with teachers in Indonesia and Lebanon in 2023.

The Staff Peer Support Groups are not a stand-alone program because they are intended to complement and diversify existing staff well-being initiatives and are also not intended to replace staff access to professional mental health counseling and other more focused services available to staff through employee assistance programs and policies.

Two Ways That HEART Provides Arts-Based Psychosocial Support to Staff

HEART provides arts-based psychosocial support to staff through two main approaches: through experiential training of facilitators for the standard program with children and through the Staff Peer Support Group Program.

Experiential Training of HEART Facilitators

HEART provides arts-based psychosocial support for staff through the standard HEART program for children because the training for HEART facilitators (4.5-day introductory training and two-day refresher training) is an experiential training process in which participants (staff) engage in HEART sessions with their peers and then discuss methods for integrating the program into their work with children. Staff engage in creative self-expression, play-based communication, and supportive group communication throughout the training. Through this process, they focus on their own well-being and bond with their peers. Because many training participants often come from the same work environment, such as a school, the bonding and social connection that develop during the HEART training is likely to continue post-training once they return to work and support each other to use the program with children. Follow-up mentoring, program-monitoring activities, and reflective consultations with Save the Children HEART staff provide additional opportunities for supportive communication, in addition to refresher training and other local events that promote the program within communities.

For many adult participants, the supportive nature of HEART training is the first time in their lives that they have been exposed to structured psychosocial support activities. By participating in the training program, they have an opportunity to share, listen, express, and process their experiences and feelings in an emotionally safe, nonjudgmental, and compassionate environment.

In a 2023 global survey of HEART training participation experience, respondents reported increased awareness of their own personal well-being and improved prioritization of self-care after participating in training sessions. Staff shared that participating in HEART training offered them opportunities to feel refreshed, relaxed, calm, and mindful and that the process provided them a space to process stress. Some also shared that they felt better able to communicate with others, experienced the development of trust among colleagues they did not know well before the training, and increased confidence in exploring their own artistic identity (Save the Children, 2023a).

> I was able to take a step back from my usual mentality of "there is so much I need to do" and focus instead on what is impacting me and how. It was a great exercise in mindfulness.
>
> (HEART Training Participant)

Multiple respondents also shared that HEART activities or techniques have become a regular part of their lives outside of work because they use them at home with their own children or with themselves when feeling stressed.

When asked to describe memorable or impactful experiences while leading HEART trainings as trainers, respondents shared experiences of witnessing adult participants become comfortable sharing their feelings and engaged in listening to others and sharing experiences. Staff also reflected on feedback they received from other HEART facilitators after implementing the program with children and shared that facilitators often express a sense of bonding with other colleagues, a positive influence on personal relationships, and a sense of fulfilment from meaningful work and that facilitators often share that "they want more trainings like this" (Save the Children, 2023a).

Another consistent observation is that during and after HEART trainings worldwide, participants stay in close contact with the training group, forming informal peer support networks. These networks not only support ongoing professional development by improving communication and collaboration among colleagues but also create new friendships that extend within and beyond the workplace (Save the Children, 2023a).

At a minimum, every HEART facilitator experiences direct psychosocial support through participation in the experiential training process, including the introductory training and refresher training. The monitoring process also aims to be supportive, with Save the Children staff helping facilitators to address challenges in constructive ways through regular program-monitoring visits (often monthly or quarterly). Many country teams also organize quarterly or annual HEART consultation meetings with facilitators, which also serve to enable a supportive community of colleagues often working in similarly stressful conditions and to organize platforms for remote communication between these face-to-face events, including e-mail groups, online closed social media groups, and group messaging mechanisms, so that a community of practice is able to maintain regular communication throughout the year to support each other to address challenges and celebrate successes.

Staff Peer Support Groups

HEART provides arts-based psychosocial support to staff through the Staff Peer Support Group Program through which staff attend regular peer support group meetings that are facilitated by trained staff/colleagues over an extended period of time. Similar to the Parent and Caregiver Peer Support Groups, the Staff Peer Support Groups are set up in phases. This program consists of weekly or biweekly structured sessions of 90 minutes each, in groups of eight to 15 participants. Each structured session includes mindfulness and relaxation activities, expressive drawing or writing on a specific topic or theme, a sharing and support circle, a grounding activity, and a self-care reflection[2] and self-care homework. Additionally, chat-and-connect sessions can be added regularly or on an ad hoc basis. The chat-and-connect sessions are mainly open discussion opportunities where no specific theme is discussed, but participants and facilitators simply share anything on their minds, and the discussion flows as needed. These open discussion sessions can start with a short relaxation activity and end with a grounding activity or a self-care reflection/commitment and can be as short as 30 minutes or as long as a standard 90-minute session.

The goal of the program is to provide long-term psychosocial support in multiple phases. The program can run over an extended period, starting with eight structured sessions in its first phase. Depending on the context and the needs of the participants, the program can be extended to a second and a third phase should participants choose to continue with their groups. In the last two phases, participants decide the frequency, regularity, and duration of sessions and whether they are structured or chat-and-connect sessions or a mixture of both. The sessions are

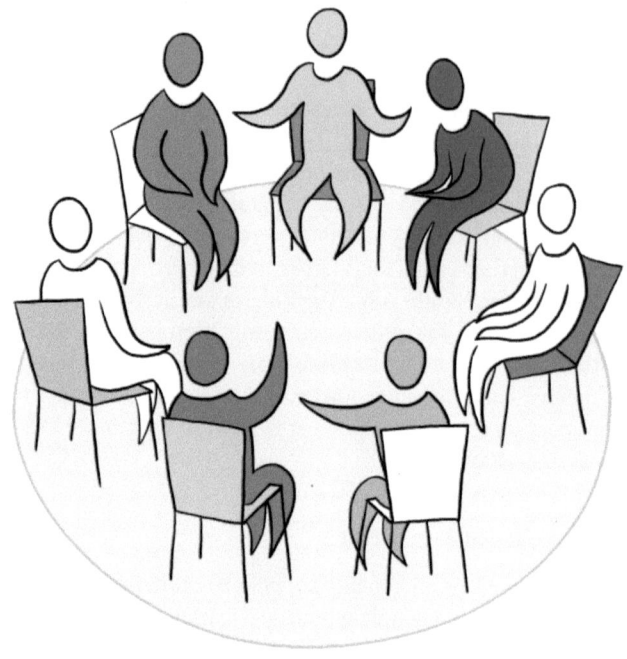

Figure 9.1 Staff peer support group set-up
Source: Kristyn S. Stickley

led by two facilitators. All facilitators attend a three-day training program, complemented with a refresher training session after three months of implementation. In addition, facilitators attend regular group supervision sessions with an experienced mental health supervisor. Facilitators are sometimes Save the Children staff members or partner NGO staff members. They are also community support workers such as community social workers or community health workers or school-based support staff such as teachers or school counselors.

Experiences of the first pilot of the program, through remote video facilitation for Save the Children employees in the United States during the COVID-19 lockdown in 2020, produced the extremely positive results that encouraged the global adaptation of the program, eventually leading to new program pilots in Lebanon and Indonesia.

Save the Children Employee (United States)

I participated in the remote peer support program during the COVID-19 lock down (sic) that brought together a disparate group of staff from different departments within Save the Children to support each other during a period of intense stress both personal and work-related. I was profoundly amazed that this organization dedicated resources to helping its staff engage with one another and build and maintain community during this period of intense stress. During COVID-19 (and after) this group has been a virtual lifeline that enabled me to continue to maximize my contributions to the important work we were doing without burning out. We are spread across the country with one member in the United Kingdom and have only ever met virtually, but we were able to establish a virtual community that helped me to rally around organizational goals and objectives while also prioritizing my own well-being. Through the exercises we shared together, we formed a bond that allowed each of us to be authentic and vulnerable while we dug deep to find the strength to persevere.

(Save the Children, 2023d)

Save the Children Employee (United States)

In the early stages, the Staff Peer Support Group was an invaluable opportunity to connect with colleagues and engage in activities to support my mental health at an incredibly challenging time. Like so many people, the pandemic upended my entire life. My household was comprised of a 15-month-old child as well as my parents, who were within the high-risk category. My mom has early onset Alzheimer's, so it was extremely stressful to think about how to keep her safe and limit our exposure. My husband made the very difficult decision to temporarily close his small business to reduce the risk of exposure for our household and we pulled our son out of daycare (sic). It was a very stressful time. This group gave me a sense of stability, community, and purpose and has since blossomed into a deep and trusting friendship. It has become one of the most rewarding experiences of my career at Save the Children. Our mission at Save the Children requires so much dedication, but it also requires staff to prioritize their own well-being to avoid burnout and to promote engagement and retention. Through our meetings, I have learned real and lasting techniques for self-care and developed a strong community of support.

(Save the Children, 2023d)

Staff Peer Support Groups in Indonesia

The Staff Peer Support Group Program was piloted in Indonesia in 2021. Indonesia is prone to natural disasters including floods, landslides, volcanic eruptions, and extreme weather, all of which serve as significant stressors for communities. The need for multilayered approaches to staff well-being is great, especially low-cost program models that can integrate into existing workspaces, utilize local facilitators, and sustain themselves over time.

During the COVID-19 pandemic, health-care workers were under tremendous pressure to keep delivering health-care to the general population while also coping with lockdown and movement restrictions, and personal stressors. Their work included supporting testing, vaccinations, and treatment of COVID-19 patients while managing personal exposure to infection and dealing with the stigma of working in high-exposure settings, and managing their own psychosocial well-being (Save the Children, 2022b). Health-care workers experienced high levels of stress, sleep deprivation and disturbance, loss of appetite, anxiety, and depressive symptoms (Save the Children, 2022b). Teachers also faced increased stressors due to the adoption of distance learning, which brought with it difficulty accessing resources, technical barriers, and reduced student participation, particularly in rural schools where high-speed internet was unavailable and students lacked the electronic devices needed to connect to school remotely (Churiyah et al., 2020; Rasmitadila et al., 2020). These challenges led to increased feelings of stress, confusion, and frustration for students, teachers, and parents (Churiyah et al., 2020; Rasmitadila et al., 2020). It was within this context that Save the Children began supporting government efforts to increase psychosocial well-being for community health workers and teachers.

Save the Children Indonesia, together with NGO partners, implements a multilayered Mental Health and Psychosocial Support (MHPSS) program for children and families. The goal of the project is to strengthen MHPSS programs and services in public schools, government-mandated community health clinics (*puskesmas*), and community-based centers. This goal includes a specific focus on supporting the psychosocial well-being of staff from Save the Children and implementing partner NGOs, schools, and community health clinics.

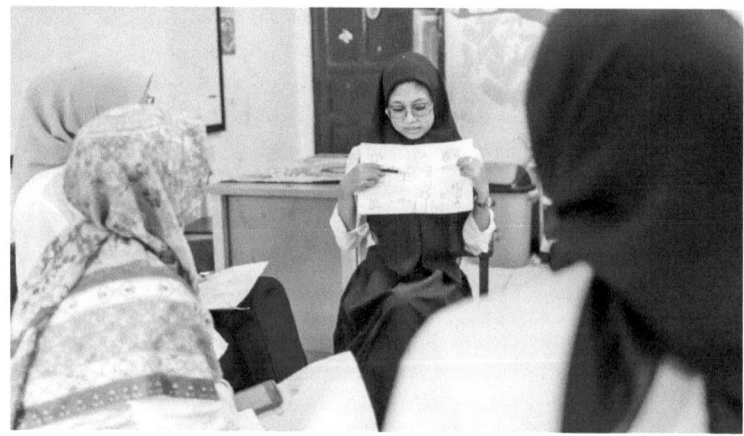

Figure 9.2 Teachers participate in HEART-adapted staff peer support group in Indonesia

Source: Save the Children

During the 2021–2022 period, the Staff Peer Support Group pilot reached a total of 25 Save the Children and partner NGO staff members, 75 teachers, and 20 health-care workers from two community health clinics. Each of these groups shared common stressors such as those related to responding to the COVID-19 pandemic but also unique stressors inherent in each profession and in individual life experiences. The Staff Peer Support Group pilots in Indonesia were organized and conducted primarily online in 2021 and 2022, and a feedback survey was conducted at the end of phase 1 (after the completion of the first eight sessions). In 2023, the Staff Peer Support Group Program expanded to support more teachers in schools through a face-to-face program model.

The survey conducted after the first phase of the pilot provided participants with an opportunity to share feedback on their overall experience participating in the Staff Peer Support Groups. The questions surveyed the level of participant satisfaction with the program, collected feedback on program logistics and content such as the scheduling and duration of sessions along with activity and discussion topics, and collected participant reflections on how the program impacted their well-being.

Participants were asked about the most common challenges they experienced related to their participation in the groups. The most reported challenge was in relation to work or personal obligations that prevented regular participation. This issue was strongest among health-care workers, 55% of whom indicated that work obligations created barriers to regular participation. Given the complex working environment for health workers during COVID-19, this result is not surprising. It is important for staff to have appropriate time and space during their workdays to slow down, take care of their own needs, and process the stress they are experiencing. The more recent 2023 in-person Staff Peer Support Group programming for teachers in Indonesia has experienced fewer challenges related to participant participation (than the health workers during the initial pilot), most likely because the sessions are organized at the school, during or after the school day, at a time that is convenient for all group members.

Three specific questions related to the program's impact on the subjective well-being of participants were asked, including the impact that participation in the program had on mood, self-care routines, and feelings of social connectedness. In the survey, responses to these three areas were collected using a 5-point Likert scale that allowed for responses that included very positive, positive, neutral, negative, or very negative. As seen in the figures below, the survey results demonstrated mostly positive or very positive outcomes for all three indicators.

Positive Impact on Mood in Indonesia

In Indonesia, 42% of teacher participants reported that their participation in the peer support groups resulted in a very positive and 53% reported a positive, impact on their mood. A total of 5% of teacher respondents in Indonesia had a

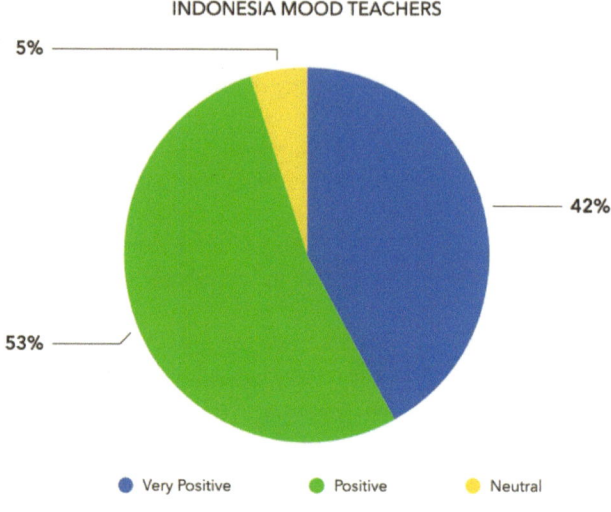

Figure 9.3 Impact on mood for teachers in Indonesia

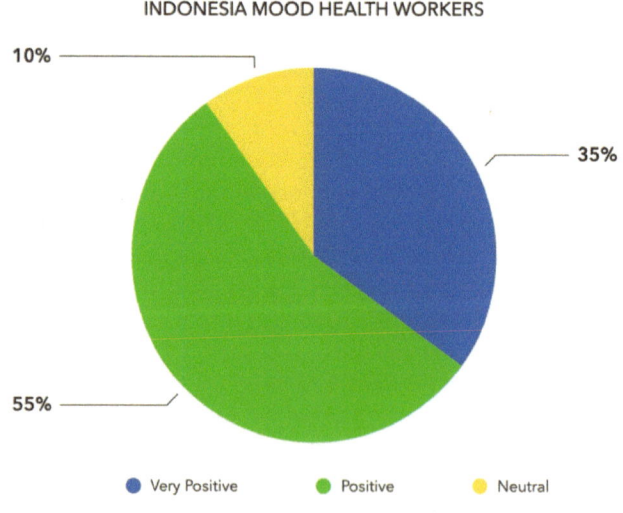

Figure 9.4 Impact on mood for health-care workers in Indonesia

neutral response (no impact, either positive or negative). For health-care workers, 35% of respondents reported a very positive impact on mood, with 55% reporting a positive impact and 10% a neutral impact.

Positive Impact on Social Connectedness in Indonesia

In Indonesia, 32% of teachers surveyed reported a very positive and 59% reported a positive impact on social connectedness, with 9% neutral. For health workers, 30% of respondents reported a very positive impact on social connectedness; 45% reported a positive impact; and 25% provided a neutral response.

Positive Impact on Self-Care Routine in Indonesia

In Indonesia, 34% of teachers reported that participating in the program had a very positive impact on their self-care routine, with 58% reporting a positive impact and 8% neutral. For health workers, 25% of participants surveyed reported a very positive, and 55% a positive, impact on self-care routine, with 20% reporting a neutral response.

More research is needed to understand the unique experiences of individuals as well as the differences in experiences among the health workers and teachers who participated in the pilots of the Staff Peer Support Groups in Indonesia. The

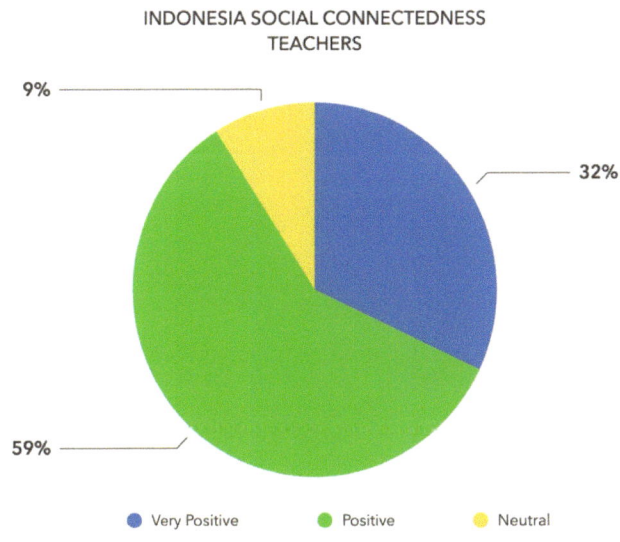

Figure 9.5 Impact on Social Connectedness for Teachers in Indonesia

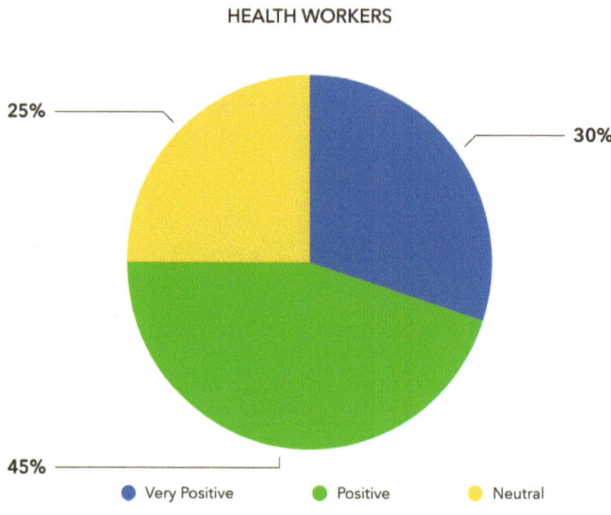

Figure 9.6 Impact on Social Connectedness for Health-Care Workers in Indonesia

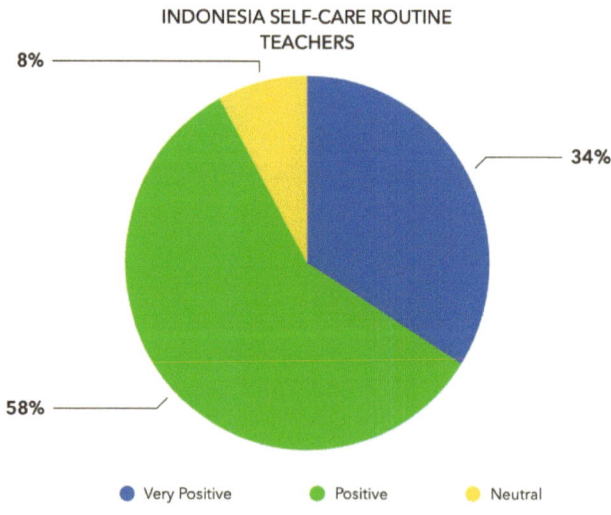

Figure 9.7 Impact on self-care routine on teachers in Indonesia

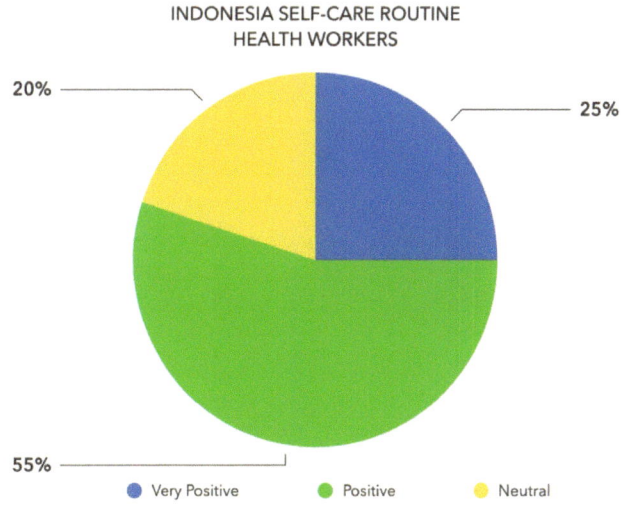

Figure 9.8 Impact on self-care routine on health-care workers in Indonesia

specific experiences of these two distinct workforces at the time of the intervention are important to consider (during the height of the COVID-19 pandemic). It is also important to compare staff experiences during the first pilots (2021–2022), which were mostly facilitated through remote video meetings, to the more recent Teacher Peer Support Groups that began in 2023 using in-person meetings. The details of staff experiences based on time, location, and specific contextual operational stressors are important to consider when comparing staff experiences across different settings, as are the ways in which the program adapts to different programming contexts and needs.

Discussion

Staff is referred to as a broad concept in this chapter. To provide more tailored support services, additional research is needed to understand the unique needs of specific staff communities within the global development and humanitarian response communities—whether they be health-care providers, teachers, or humanitarian organization staff. Understanding the daily work demands of different groups is as important as understanding the needs of the children, families, and communities that humanitarian workers serve. Staffing and managerial models designed to support staff well-being as part of the workday will need dedicated time for problem solving to address common obstacles—for example, heavy workloads that prevent participation. A shift toward staff care during work hours will require scheduling, staffing, and work schedule adjustments along with other site-specific adaptations that will allow staff to briefly disengage from their more traditional responsibilities to prioritize their own mental health and psychosocial well-being.

Key to the approach of HEART training in general, and Staff Peer Support Groups in particular, is the importance of human connection. Expanding staff well-being programs grounded in social support, expressive arts, compassion, and empathy in global development and humanitarian response programming can have a ripple effect in supporting staff longevity within organizations, and this ripple effect can only benefit the children, families, and communities that such organizations support. We hope this chapter will inspire more agencies to develop policies and practices that incorporate multiple and diverse wellness modalities for their staff and partners. Approaches can be adapted to resonate more closely with specific cultural contexts to reduce burnout, enhance social connections, and provide a space to process stress through supportive communication. Additional research could also explore how such approaches support staff retention, work quality, and cost savings related to staff well-being outcomes.

Conclusion

As operational stress levels associated with humanitarian response and international development work continue to increase in the face of natural and human-made disasters, there is also a growing awareness of the pitfalls and dangers of staff stress and burnout. Staff working in highly stressful environments require MHPSS to ensure their ability to cope and recover from operational stressors related to working in contexts of adversity or in work environments with regular exposure to human suffering. Arts-based psychosocial support approaches for staff well-being are effective and low-cost options for integrating effective staff well-being support into diverse working environments within the global development and humanitarian response sectors. The experience of the HEART program in supporting staff well-being provides a practical example of how arts-based group psychosocial support can improve staff well-being in different working environments around the world.

Key Takeaways

- Staff working in global development and humanitarian response experience unique stressors related to working in conditions of adversity.
- Participation in experiential HEART training offers an opportunity for staff to engage directly in arts-based psychosocial support and has been linked to improved staff well-being.

- HEART-adapted Staff Peer Support Groups offer an opportunity for enhanced staff well-being through organized and facilitated creative expression and supportive communication and have demonstrated improved well-being among participants.

Notes

1 The program is intended to be facilitated face to face but can be adapted to a remote video facilitation method if in-person group meetings are not possible and appropriate technological support is available to ensure quality video facilitation (electricity, Wi-Fi, and relevant technological equipment).
2 The topic of self-care is addressed repeatedly throughout the first phase of the support group program. At the end of each support group session, a homework assignment is given to the participants to practice some type of self-care every day. Reflections on self-care take place regularly with a focus on intentional planning for practical ways to do things every day that promote relaxation and stress processing.

Chapter 10

Scaling of Healing and Education Through the Arts in Collaboration with Local Partners

Sara Hommel, Ana Lagidze, and Miroslava Marjanovic

Introduction

Scaling is generally accepted to mean expansion. For the sake of this discussion on scaling Healing and Education Through the Arts (HEART), we consider scaling to be the process of expanding HEART to reach more people and recognize that scaling goals differ from one context and location to another. Successful scaling is dependent on program quality, fidelity, and sustainability. It is important to note that scaling goals can include expanding programming to reach an entire population or specific sections of the population distinguished by age, geographic location, exposure to specific contexts of adversity, or enrollment in or engagement with, a specific space through which HEART is delivered, such as a school or community-based service location. As such, the case examples shared in this chapter demonstrate different methods of scaling with varied scaling goals provided in each example.

The experience of scaling HEART in different countries and contexts has produced several key observations on success factors for scaling with quality, fidelity, and sustainability. Successful HEART scaling requires providing stakeholder partnerships with clear expectations and obligations, setting up effective coordination mechanisms among relevant stakeholders, establishing long-term funding commitments, providing quality training mechanisms that are sustainably staffed by relevant partner institutions, programming fidelity commitments including staffing and supplies within dedicated spaces such as classrooms or centers, and post-scaling stakeholder commitments to ensure sustainability at scale.

Scaling Child Support Programming in Complex Settings

Scaling arts-based psychosocial support programming for children, families, and communities in conditions of adversity involves the coordination of multiple actors in complex operational environments that intersect with local and

DOI: 10.4324/9781003367529-11

national stakeholders across the public health, educational, and social welfare sectors.

Complex systems can be a threat to scaling, particularly when fragmented across multiple domains of child and family support services (Gupta et al., 2021). When scaling a child and family support approach in a complex system that relies on para-professional or nonspecialized facilitators, staff turnover can pose a threat to successful scaling or the sustainability of programming at scale. This situation is particularly relevant in contexts where the involved workforce is underpaid and/or undertrained (Gupta et al., 2021). The experience of scaling HEART in preschool settings has been particularly challenging in contexts with under-professionalized early childhood educational settings.

Sustaining a quality workforce not only requires quality training, supervision, and infrastructure, it also requires investment in the well-being of staff (Pacchiano et al., 2021). Recognizing and rewarding good work and ensuring support for the psychosocial needs of the workforce can ensure greater job satisfaction that results in staff retention and sustainable quality programming before, during, and after scaling.

Successful scaling is dependent on the quality of program administration and the continuity of key aspects of that quality over time. These goals include sustained quality training of the workforce supported by stable and strong infrastructure, which enables quality supervision over time, which serves to maintain program fidelity (Caron, Bernard, & Metz, 2021). Program fidelity for HEART scaling is necessary to ensure program impact at scale and requires intentional planning, monitoring, and problem-solving strategies both throughout the scaling process and once scaling is complete. Partnerships with local training institutions or professional associations that support preservice and in-service training of child support professionals is critical for sustaining program quality and fidelity at scale. Also critical are long-term funding commitments from local stakeholders and strong coordination between funding stakeholders and those responsible for training, monitoring, and ensuring quality programming.

Commitments and collaborations among multiple stakeholders within complex scaling environments require the coordination of policy makers, government agencies, donors, researchers, practitioners, and local, regional, or global organizations (Carter et al., 2021). In the experience of HEART, relevant organizations often include Save the Children, local nongovernmental organizations, national associations, and interorganizational groups that support local or regional stakeholder coordination (interorganizational coordination groups might exist before scaling or might need to be created specifically for HEART scaling). Strong coordination mechanisms that hold individual stakeholders to individual and group commitments are necessary both during the scaling process and once scale is reached, to ensure that program quality and fidelity are sustained at scale.

Funding for scaling often centers on costs associated with training facilitators, supplying classrooms or centers with arts materials, supporting program monitoring mechanisms, and sustaining post-scaling costs including refresher trainings for existing staff, training of new staff when they enter the workforce, restocking of classrooms and centers with arts materials, and staffing coordination mechanisms (dedicated staff time from relevant stakeholder groups). Long-term funding commitments that are flexible and support stakeholders to adapt to changing programming needs along the scaling process are particularly helpful when scaling child support programming in complex settings where children, families, and communities are affected by multiple adversities. The scaling experience of HEART has highlighted the need for locally designed flexible scaling strategies that support unique challenges and opportunities in the local setting and allow for the process to adapt and change over time.

Adaptation Within a Scaling Context

Some countries experience a transition between different stages of humanitarian response and development programming over extended periods of time. For example, long-term humanitarian response settings such as those that support refugees or internally displaced persons can experience different stages of program delivery logistics, financing, staffing, and community participation at different points in time over many years. Within a framework of scaling or sustaining with quality at scale, a program such as HEART needs to be able to adapt to the constantly changing environment. An example is the use of the program in Ukraine over the last decade. HEART first began in Ukraine in 2014 as part of a response to support internally displaced children and families. The program was initially used in preschools, primary schools, and community centers in central and eastern Ukraine, in areas with high populations of internally displaced persons who fled armed conflict in the Donetsk Oblast region of southeastern Ukraine. In 2020 and 2021, during the COVID-19 lockdown, when schools and community centers were closed, HEART in Ukraine transitioned to a home support model through which bags of arts supplies were delivered to children and families at home, along with a short pamphlet to guide parents and caregivers on simple expressive arts activities to do with their children. In 2022, when the most recent conflict started, HEART began a new phase of adaptation that started with the use of the HEART at Home model to support children in shelters across different regions of Ukraine (often underground shelters used to keep children and families safe during bombings). Once it was safe for children to return to schools or community centers, in some areas of the country, a condensed version[1] of HEART (approximately 20% of the program) was used by existing HEART facilitators and newly trained facilitators (training of new facilitators started in 2023 to expand the program to new regions). The Condensed

HEART program continued to expand to support children in preschools, primary schools, and community centers in different parts of the country in early 2024, with plans to transition to the full program when appropriate in the future. In this type of transitionary program model, scaling is specific to time and location and the program model adapts to what is needed and possible when, where, and how.

Financing for Scaling Healing and Education Through the Arts

The complex funding environments of global development and humanitarian response settings pose unique challenges for scaling up and sustaining arts-based psychosocial support. Complex multisectoral policy and programming environments with fragmented funding mechanisms often lack pre-existing coordination mechanisms. For an organization leading a scaling process, funding coordination demands multiyear planning with sustainable funding commitments. Both humanitarian response and global development programming can include funding from multilateral and bilateral donor agencies, private donors such as foundations, local government agencies, and others. For HEART, two key aspects of financial planning and coordination have been key to successful scaling. These include sustainable and flexible funding support from private foundations and sustainable funding commitments from local government agencies.

In humanitarian response settings, sustainable and flexible funding support from private foundations has been used to supplement complex multisectoral bilateral or multilateral donor financing, which has ensured the sustainability of quality programming at whatever scale is deemed appropriate for a specific time and location. Such contexts often include temporary programming, depending on the emergency they respond to (such as conflict, displacement, or natural disaster). These locations eventually transition to something else after an initial emergency response period, and flexible private donor funding has ensured the ability of HEART to adapt and transition to meet local contextual needs during post-emergency recovery programming or transition from humanitarian response to development programming over time.

In global development settings, funding for scaling is dependent on local policy makers and government agencies because the scaling is intended to be permanent through integration into sustainable local child support settings financed by public agencies or institutions. Funding from private foundations is often used to supplement the HEART scaling process alongside funding from local stakeholders, but once scale is reached, sustainability of quality HEART programming at scale is dependent on long-term funding within the systems or sectors where HEART integration has successfully scaled, such as the national, provincial, or municipal education systems.

Flexible private funding that supplements public budgets throughout the scaling process is important to allow Save the Children to support local partners to adapt to meet changing local needs, but sustaining HEART once scale is reached is only possible when program sustainability costs are fully integrated into public sector budgets. Private donors and foundations have supported the HEART scaling process in several different countries. Some provided financial support for one year, contributing to a specific time and place of the HEART scaling process in one country, whereas others have supported HEART scaling over several years, supporting different stages of the scaling process at different times. The complex process of coordinating funding commitments across multiple partners requires a focused approach that does not rush the scaling process but rather scales step-by-step across programming locations and ensures appropriate funding for all aspects of program expansion. This approach might require slowing down at certain moments within the scaling process, because program quality and fidelity are priorities. The flexible multiyear private funding that supports a process of local adaptation, piloting, revision, standardization, and step-by-step scaling over time has been the most significant component of successful HEART scaling globally because it has allowed Save the Children to supplement the funding commitments of local partners to ensure program quality, fidelity, and sustainability.

Healing and Education Through the Arts Champions within Scaling Strategies

It is important to have advocacy champions within all relevant stakeholder groups including practitioners, donors, policy makers, and others. Within HEART scaling experiences, key advocacy champions have played strategic roles in building understanding, spreading knowledge, and coordinating commitments of their respective stakeholder groups. Of particular importance for HEART scaling have been advocacy champions including donors, policy makers, teachers, parents, and children. When those receiving the program, delivering the program, funding the program, and coordinating the program all feel respected and valued as key stakeholders within a complex system, scaling with quality, fidelity, and sustainability is possible.

Conditions for Successful Scaling of Healing and Education Through the Arts

The experience of scaling HEART in different settings across multiple countries has highlighted several key conditions for scaling success. Advocacy champions within local stakeholder groups are imperative as is evidence that can inform stakeholder decision making and scaling commitments. Evidence that clarifies what is needed to ensure program quality ensures that stakeholders have the knowledge needed to make informed commitments that ensure program fidelity and sustainability.

Conditions for successful scaling commitments rely on appropriate funding during the scaling process and funding for sustainability of quality programming once scale is reached, which requires clear agreements among stakeholders related to funding commitments throughout and after scaling. Clear partnership agreements extend beyond funding because they also clarify the roles and responsibilities of partners, and such partnership agreements require strong coordination mechanisms to ensure those responsibilities are met. Within partnership agreements and funding commitments, flexibility is necessary to adapt the scaling process to meet changing local needs and challenges, and this goal requires a scaling plan that is not rushed and allows for coordination, communication, and action for problem solving and scaling process adaptation as needed. Scaling HEART in complex systems is possible when clear partnership commitments are well coordinated and designed to adapt and evolve to ensure quality, fidelity, and sustainability.

Experiences Scaling Healing and Education Through the Arts

Scaling Healing and Education Through the Arts in Primary Schools in Bosnia and Herzegovina

HEART was first piloted in Bosnia and Herzegovina in 2014. Over the course of four years, from 2014 to 2017, the program was piloted in different settings (preschools, primary schools, community centers, and disability support programs) in several different areas of the country. This experience varied over several years and tested the program in a range of settings with different levels of local stakeholder commitments, allowing the national Save the Children office in Bosnia and Herzegovina to identify locally effective conditions for scaling and then to focus time, funding, and coordination on a specific location with a high level of multistakeholder commitment to scaling and sustaining the program. In 2018, a HEART scaling process started in Una Sana Canton (geographic district in the northwest part of the country), aimed at integrating HEART into all primary schools in the district.

Planning for scaling HEART in Una Sana Canton started after a series of introductory HEART trainings for teachers and school counselors. The goal of the local model was to train school counselors in addition to teachers so that the school counselors could serve as co-facilitators to support teachers with large classes. The school counselors were also able to integrate expressive arts methods into their individual and group counseling work in the schools. When the response was positive, and more teachers and school counselors in the district requested training, Save the Children invited school administrators to join the next round of training, so they could experience the program firsthand alongside their staff. The positive reaction of the school administrators led to the designation of "HEART Friendly Schools," which were set up as centers of excellence for HEART, and to the design of the first phase of a district-wide scaling strategy. Within the first phase of the scaling strategy, a goal was set to train all teachers and school counselors within the HEART Friendly Schools to serve as advocacy champions for other schools in the district throughout the scaling process.

As word spread about the HEART Friendly Schools, increasing numbers of teachers and administrators from other schools from across the district contacted Save the Children to request support for integrating HEART into their schools. Over the next several years, Save the Children trained all the teachers and counselors within the HEART Friendly Schools and then trained and mentored a number of those teachers and counselors as HEART trainers, to be able to train others in schools throughout the district. The first phase of HEART in each school included Save the Children-coordinated and -funded training of teachers and counselors, post-training program monitoring and mentoring from Save the Children, and arts materials for classrooms. School Action Plans (SAPs) were designed by the HEART Friendly Schools to incorporate HEART into the regular school curricula and extracurricular activities, and these SAPs were approved by the school boards. In addition, the Ministry of Education (MoE) agreed to integrate the cost of arts materials into the school budget after the first year of Save the Children support (funding for arts materials and training teachers and school counselors).

In parallel to the first phase of HEART expansion in HEART Friendly Schools, Save the Children worked closely with the local educational authorities including the MoE of Una Sana Canton to identify, document, and implement a best practices strategy to ensure the sustainability of the HEART program in all Una Sana primary schools beyond the initial scaling. Building on the success of the formalized integration of the SAP program into the HEART Friendly Schools, a process was organized to support all schools to identify appropriate times for HEART sessions both within and beyond the school day. A review of the existing district-wide primary school curricula was undertaken to identify how specific HEART sessions linked with key mandatory topics within the primary school curricula. This step led to the design of a locally customized Guidance Note that highlighted logistical and content-specific approaches to HEART integration, including how HEART sessions can be organized within existing subject-specific lesson times where specific HEART session topics or goals overlap with those of the formal curricula.[2]

The Guidance Note for HEART integration into the primary school curricula was launched in 2019 and consists of two parts. The first section explains the theoretical background of HEART, the role of the teacher as a HEART facilitator, how to adapt HEART for children with disabilities, and how the program benefits children. The benefits for children include how HEART sessions support the psychosocial well-being, learning, and development of children and how to link HEART sessions with learning outcome goals within the primary school curricula. The second part of the guidance includes 27 examples of lesson plans for different subjects within the formal curricula (three examples for each school grade level) to help teachers to identify time for HEART sessions within their weekly and monthly lesson planning throughout the school year. This approach supports teachers at all primary school grade levels to identify time within the school day for HEART.

After the completion of the new curricula integration guidance and the ongoing success of the program within the HEART Friendly Schools, a conference was organized in 2019 to bring together school and MoE representatives from across the district and across the country. The conference included presentations on program integration from the HEART Friendly Schools and break-out sessions where representatives from different schools and government offices could meet with HEART Champions from the HEART Friendly Schools to ask questions and discuss the program in more detail. The conference also included the facilitation of several HEART sessions so that participants could experience the program firsthand. The conference increased communication and coordination between multiple stakeholder groups within the district and across the country, leading to new partnerships within the next phase of scaling.

In 2021, a total of 16 teachers from HEART Friendly Schools were selected to be coached as HEART trainers to transition the process of HEART scaling to local stakeholders. As a result, by the end of 2022, the HEART scaling process in the district transitioned from being mostly led by Save the Children to being mostly led by local stakeholders. Save the Children continues to fund training and arts supplies for schools, but trainings are now mostly led by local HEART Champions. Once participants from the school are fully trained and the school receives one year of support from Save the Children, it should be able to sustain HEART with its existing budget (provided by the MoE).

Following the success of the conference and the continued scaling of HEART in primary schools across the district, Save the Children organized a series of consultations with the district's Pedagogical Faculty (the department within the local university that is responsible for training teachers and school counselors). The Vice Dean of the department attended a local HEART training program, after which the department organized a Technical Working Group, made up of faculty members, Save the Children HEART focal points, and other local HEART Champions, to design a new HEART course at the university. The new course, called "Emotional Pedagogy," is planned to start in the 2024–2025 academic year, to be offered to university students planning careers in education (teaching or school counseling). The integration of a HEART course into the academic

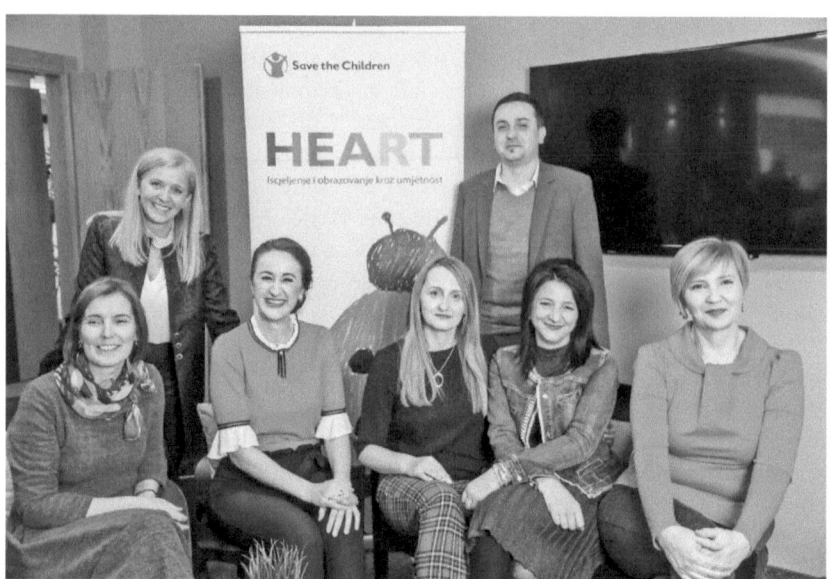

Figure 10.1 HEART champions at the conference in Bosnia and Herzegovina
Source: Save the Children

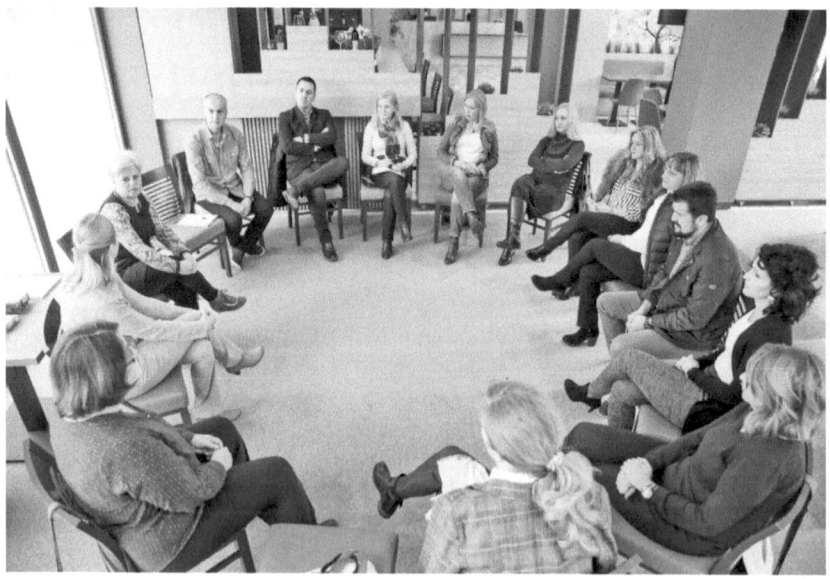

Figure 10.2 Break-out session at the HEART conference in Bosnia and Herzegovina
Source: Save the Children

department responsible for teacher training ensures that, once scaling is complete in the district, it will be sustainable through continued preservice training because all new teachers and school counselors will have it as an optional course during their formal training at the university. Thus, this course ensures that the cost of sustaining HEART at scale will be covered by local stakeholders because the MoE has integrated the cost of arts supplies into school budgets, and new teachers and school counselors will receive HEART training during their university studies.

Throughout the planned scaling process, several challenges emerged that led to a slowdown in scaling. In 2020 and 2021, scaling slowed due to COVID-19, and this slowdown continued in 2022 and 2023 as Save the Children struggled to catch up with multiple school support commitments that were postponed due to COVID-19 (including and beyond HEART). Further complications due to staff turnover, both at Save the Children and local partners, caused additional slowdown in the scaling process. The current timeline anticipates that the scaling of HEART in primary schools in Una Sana Canton should be completed in 2026, two years later than originally planned.

The experience of scaling HEART in Una Sana Canton identified the following key aspects of a successful scaling strategy: (i) the flexibility to respond to local needs (e.g. development of HEART Guidance for curricula integration); (ii) advocacy opportunities for local HEART Champions (HEART Conference); (iii) support from policy makers or policy institutions (e.g. Ministry of Education); (iv) local capacity for scaling (e.g. 16 Local HEART Trainers); (v) long-term sustainable capacity strengthening support (e.g. Pedagogical Faculty HEART course); (vi) financing for sustainability at scale (e.g. program costs integrated into school budgets); and (vii) local demand from primary school administrations, teachers, and children (e.g. HEART Friendly Schools as an example of program excellence).

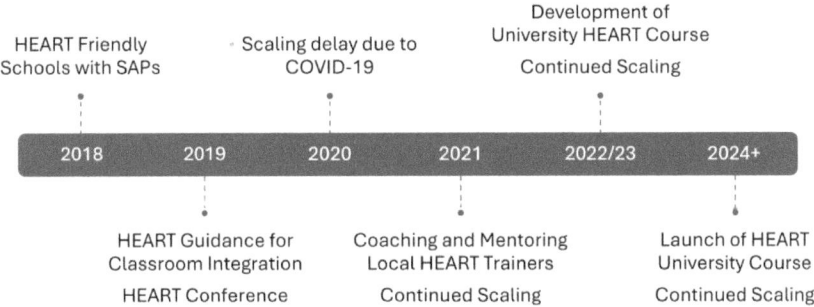

Figure 10.3 Timeline for scaling HEART in Una Sana Canton, Bosnia and Herzegovina

As of 2024, the scaling of HEART in Una Sana Canton is approximately 60% complete. The HEART University Course is expected to launch in the second half of 2024. Full scaling in the district is expected to be completed by the end of 2026, which is two years later than originally planned due to COVID-related scaling delay and slowdown.

Scaling Healing and Education Through the Arts in Preschools in Georgia

After the successful integration of HEART programs into community-based centers for children with disabilities in Georgia, Save the Children organized a series of consultations with local early-education stakeholders (e.g. Ministry of Education, National Preschool Association, Tbilisi Kindergarten Management Agency) in 2018 to plan a pilot of HEART in preschools in Tbilisi. Bringing local partners into the early stages of the pilot-planning process created a sense of shared ownership of the pilot. The partners identified 20 preschools to participate in the first pilot. In the first year of piloting, Save the Children facilitated HEART trainings for preschool teachers and representatives from the Ministry of Education's Preschool Education Division, so that the MoE could observe the process of preschool teacher professional development firsthand.

After the first year of piloting, Save the Children reviewed the program monitoring data and stakeholder feedback, and in response to increasing demand in Tbilisi and beyond, expanded the pilot to more preschools including those in both the Tbilisi and Rustavi municipalities. In 2020, COVID-19 forced preschools to close across the country, so Save the Children organized the distribution of HEART at Home[3] for children attending HEART integrated preschools. HEART at Home was so popular that the Rustavi mayor's office funded its expansion to preschools not yet participating in the pilot, to ensure that all preschool children in the city received the home support package during the COVID-19 school closure.

In 2021, amid continued school closures, Save the Children partnered with the Ministry of Education to record three HEART Session Videos that aired on the Ministry of Education television station (programming to support children's learning and development at home during COVID-19 school closures). The HEART sessions aired to a viewing audience of approximately 300,000 households with preschool age children and aimed to guide children and caregivers through expressive arts activities they could do together at home. The HEART television sessions led to an increase in local demand for the program, including from parents and children, encouraging local and national stakeholders to expand beyond the pilot programs in Tbilisi and Rustavi.

In response to growing demand for HEART expansion across the country, Save the Children partnered with the National Preschool Association to organize an advocacy event in 2021 to promote the coordination of HEART scale-up

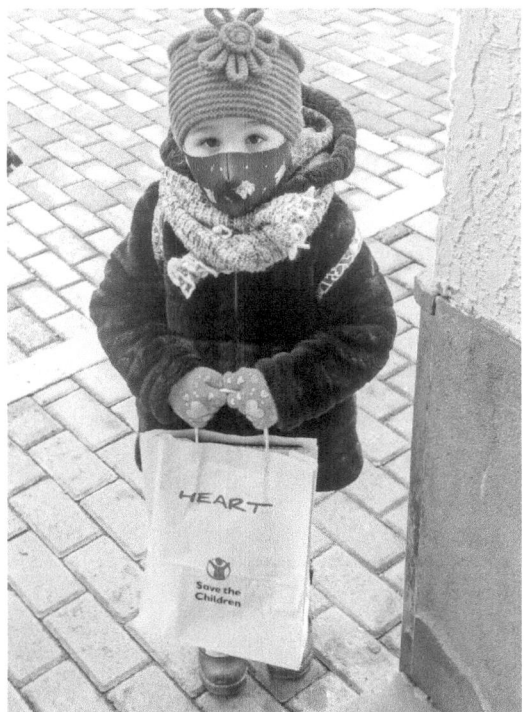

Figure 10.4 HEART at Home kit collection during COVID-19 school closure in Georgia

Source: Save the Children

among multiple partner organizations and institutions in Georgia. The event was attended by representatives from several stakeholder groups and highlighted the experience of several key HEART Advocacy Champions including teachers, MoE representatives, officials from the Tbilisi Kindergarten Management Agency, and several municipal government representatives. During the event, the Tbilisi Kindergarten Management Agency shared results from a local situational analysis conducted by the agency to identify opportunities for preschool improvement. The results identified HEART as the most requested program by teachers and parents, and specifically noted that the impact teachers shared related to how HEART provides teachers with practical methods to support children with special needs as an integrated inclusive educational approach. The agency then announced a new three-year strategy and action plan for preschool improvement based on scaling HEART to all preschools in the municipality.

In a follow-up to the event, stakeholder coordination continued to grow; in 2022, the launch of a national scaling strategy for HEART in preschools in

Georgia began. With sustainability funding from local municipal budgets (to cover the costs of sustaining HEART after the initial Save the Children-supported training, coaching, and arts supplies for classrooms), the national scale-up strategy for HEART began with a city-by-city expansion process. To expand the number of HEART trainers available for scaling, Save the Children coached and mentored experienced preschool teachers and Kindergarten Union staff as new HEART trainers. When the first pilot of HEART in preschools started in 2018, the Save the Children office in Georgia had three local HEART trainers available to train teachers. As of early 2024, there are 10 HEART trainers available to co-facilitate HEART training sessions for scaling the program across the country.

In 2022 and 2023, Save the Children in Georgia conducted several small evaluations of HEART programming in preschools. Results from the evaluations demonstrated several key impact areas including professional skills development for teachers, improved teacher attitudes toward working with children with disabilities, improved emotional regulation of children, improved social and emotional development of children, improved communication and coordination among children in the classroom, increased engagement in cooperative play among children in the classroom, and increased integration of children with disabilities in group classroom activities (Save the Children, 2021).

Results from these evaluations were integrated into consultations with partners across the country to support evidence-based policy planning. The more information policy makers have on the goals and impacts of the program, the greater is the possibility of informed decision making as to whether HEART is an approach to consider in their local municipal district and whether they are ready to take on the necessary commitments for scaling HEART.

HEART scaling in preschools in Georgia is expected to reach 80% of all preschools in Tbilisi, and 100% of all preschools in Rustavi, Kutaisi, and Bolnisi by the end of 2024. Focusing on quality training, program fidelity, and sustainable funding, the scaling strategy in Georgia requires the following commitments from local partners before HEART is integrated into a new location (municipal district):

- municipal government commitment to HEART sustainability funding after initial training and support by Save the Children (budget for arts materials and program monitoring),
- committed staff focal points with dedicated time for coordination between local partners including municipal government funding offices, kindergarten management agencies, and kindergarten unions, and
- commitment of preschools to attend training and integrate HEART into their classrooms (commitment of teachers and school administration).

By ensuring that conditions for successful scaling are met through clear agreements with local partners, the HEART scaling process prioritizes expansion based on where conditions are appropriate for scaling. This approach ensures that areas where conditions for scaling are not yet met have time to plan and develop as needed for future scaling opportunities.

Healing and Education Through the Arts Scale-up Partners in Georgia

- Ministry of Education and Science of Georgia (Preschool Education Division)
- Ministry of Education and Science of Georgia (Inclusive Education Division)
- Tbilisi Kindergarten Management Agency
- Rustavi Kindergarten Union
- Kutaisi Kindergarten Union
- Bolnisi Kindergarten Union
- Early Intervention Coalition (nongovernmental organizations and INGO Inter-Agency Coalition)
- National Center for Teacher Professional Development
- National Preschool Association

HEART Preschool Scaling Percentage Estimates by the end of 2024

- Tbilisi – 80%
- Rustavi – 100%
- Kutaisi – 100%
- Bolnisi – 100%

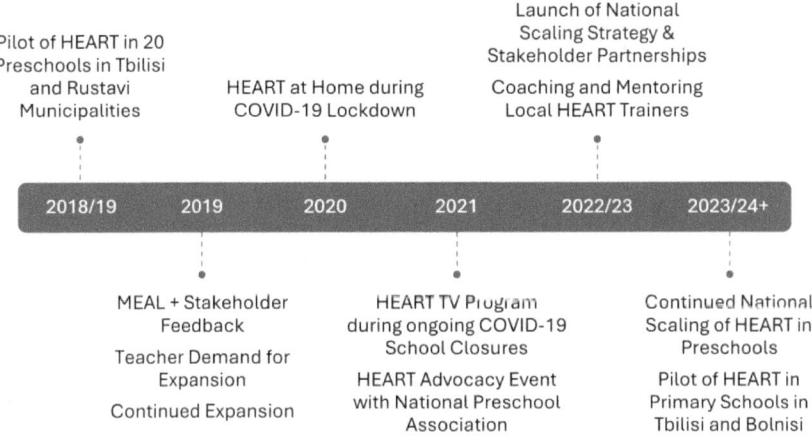

Figure 10.5 Timeline for Scaling HEART in Georgia

In 2024 and beyond, HEART scaling in Georgia will continue to complete the last 20% of scaling in Tbilisi and expand HEART to preschools in smaller cities and villages across the country. Also in 2024, Save the Children in Georgia, in partnership with the Ministry of Education, will pilot HEART in primary schools in Bolnisi and Tbilisi.

Common Elements of Successful Scaling of Healing and Education Through the Arts

The experiences of scaling HEART in Bosnia and Herzegovina and Georgia have illuminated common challenges that can threaten successful scaling and common factors that can support successful scaling. Common elements of successful scaling relate to the following specific local conditions that need to be present:

- committed funding for scaling and sustaining HEART at scale,
- skilled program staff and trainers (to train facilitators and monitor programming),
- local demand from dedicated facilitators (teachers, school counselors, and others),
- commitment to scaling with fidelity (e.g., maintain training protocols, program guidance, dosing, and arts supplies),
- HEART Champions within partner institutions and organizations,
- coordination between partners (clear roles and responsibilities in the scaling process),
- flexibility to adapt scaling processes as needed to meet local challenges along the way.

The common elements of successful HEART scaling in Georgia and in Bosnia and Herzegovina serve to guide HEART scaling plans in other countries where planning for HEART scaling is in process. The adherence to ethical programming standards and scaling processes that ensure quality, fidelity, and sustainability of HEART in Georgia and in Bosnia and Herzegovina are standards of excellence in program scaling that extend beyond HEART and can inform the scaling of child and family support programming in complex settings around the world.

Conclusion

The successful experience of scaling HEART in Georgia and in Bosnia and Herzegovina has illuminated multiple key elements to inform scaling strategies for HEART in complex environments around the world. In both countries, decisions about where to scale, when to scale, and how to scale have relied on local conditions to ensure quality scaling processes. For both countries, scaling strategies have focused on ensuring local conditions for scaling with quality, fidelity, and sustainability, and those strategies have allowed for the flexibility to adapt when needed to address challenges along the way. With quality planning, clear and committed partnerships, effective coordination, and sustainable funding, scaling arts-based psychosocial support for children in complex environments around the world is possible.

Key Takeaways

- HEART scaling experiences in Georgia and in Bosnia and Herzegovina have identified several key conditions for successful HEART scaling related to funding, staffing, stakeholder commitment, partner roles and responsibilities, coordination, and scaling process flexibility.
- HEART scaling should only take place when conditions for scaling with quality, fidelity, and sustainability are met.
- Scaling arts-based psychosocial support for children and families in complex environments is possible when stakeholder commitments ensure conditions for quality, fidelity, and sustainability.

Notes

1 Condensed HEART is an adaptation of the program designed for temporary use in unstable or transitioning environments, where the full program is not appropriate due either to logistical restrictions or the intensity of local adversity. The condensed HEART program contains approximately 20% of the full program and uses simple activities that require fewer materials and less training of facilitators. This version of the program does not include most of the structured activities that focus on specific topics and themes, because some of these topics and themes would not be appropriate during intense conditions of adversity (such as active armed conflict).

2 The guidance was particularly helpful for teachers of higher grade levels in primary schools. Often, there is more flexibility within the curriculum of lower grade levels, so early grade teachers have an easier time scheduling HEART sessions during a normal school day. The guidance helped higher grade teachers to find time for HEART sessions within a much less flexible curriculum.

3 HEART at Home includes a bag of arts supplies and a pamphlet of guidance for parents and caregivers to support the facilitation of expressive arts activities with children at home.

Chapter 11

Lessons Learned and Looking to the Future

Sara Hommel, May Aoun, Aida Bekic, and Dario Lipovac

Introduction – HEART Experiences Around the World

In previous chapters, we sought to share the complex experience of developing, adapting, and scaling a global arts-based psychosocial support program. We reviewed the theory and research that informed the design of HEART, and shared reflections on the structure and content of the program as well as the ethical standards that guide its quality. We reflected on the experience of using HEART to support children of different age groups. We discussed multiple adaptations to the program over the years including the program's adaptation to support children with disabilities, support children at home during pandemic or conflict related lockdown, support parents and caregivers, and how it adapted to support staff well-being. We also shared examples of how HEART is scaling through local partnerships in two different types of school settings (preschools and primary schools) in two different countries.

The experience of HEART is large and complex, and many lessons have been learned over the years. Several key challenges and successes of HEART have produced important learnings that inform the way the program is implemented, funded, and managed. We aim to finish by sharing some key reflections on these learnings, and on our expectations for the future of HEART.

Lessons Learned through Key Challenges

There have been many challenges during the development, adaptation, and scaling of HEART. Some have been specific to a particular time or place, an issue in a local programming context, or the complexity of a setting affected by multiple adversities. Other challenges have been experienced repeatedly, in different settings in different parts of the world, and are linked to very specific issues that have required careful attention from HEART staff and champions around the world. It is this latter category that we seek to reflect on and share key lessons learned.

DOI: 10.4324/9781003367529-12

The first global challenge is related to public perception of mental health. In many parts of the world, there is a stigma associated with mental health. Thus, the way that any Mental Health and Psychosocial Support (MHPSS) is communicated with, and delivered to, local communities, needs to be considered within a framework of what is socially appropriate or preferable in the local setting. This requires careful consideration of how psychosocial support programs, such as HEART, are named and communicated. A few lessons learned related to this challenge include:

1. Local campaigns to promote the importance of mental health for everyone can be extremely helpful as they can provide language that normalizes mental health, share information on how to access mental health support, and empower those in need to seek appropriate services and supports.
2. Clarifying the difference between specialized mental health services (clinical mental health support) and non-specialized psychosocial support (such as HEART) is often helpful in building community acceptance of a program intended for everyone.
3. Communicating the goals of HEART in ways that are understood and accepted by local communities and stakeholder groups can help clarify expectations of what the program is and how it works (including de-stigmatizing psychosocial support).[1]

The second global challenge relates to a lack of understanding of the importance of the arts in promoting psychosocial well-being, learning, and development. This requires careful attention to clarifying the design and content of the program, as well as its intended outcomes, with various stakeholders. It also requires patience with stakeholders who consider art-based approaches to be less important than other components of a holistic child support or learning environment. A few lessons learned related to this challenge include:

1. Customizing information about how arts-based approaches can support the goals of specific stakeholder groups can be very useful in building understanding and acceptance of arts-based methodologies (for example, the link between music and math or drama and language development when communicating with the education professionals).
2. Offering specific stakeholders an opportunity to participate in a HEART session, HEART training, or HEART-adapted Adult Peer Support Group, can dramatically improve understanding of how the arts can improve psychosocial well-being for people of all ages.
3. Creating opportunities for HEART Champions to share their experience of HEART within or across multiple stakeholder groups, can improve

knowledge and consideration of arts-based methodologies and increase stakeholder interest and engagement.

The third global challenge is specific to the global development and humanitarian response sectors. In recent years, we've seen a push, from some stakeholders, to reach more children at faster speed, and often without increased funding that would allow for increased staffing and supplies for program expansion. This can lead to watered-down programs in which there is less time for training child support staff, less funding of supplies for schools or centers, and shorter periods of program implementation to deliver the intended service or support to children and families. The challenge for HEART has been to reject requests for a watered-down approach, and consistently maintain its ethical programming standards. A few lessons learned related to this challenge include:

1. Inter-agency guidelines for MHPSS programming in global development and humanitarian response are helpful in supporting arguments for ethical programming standards for MHPSS.[2]
2. Advocacy within and across stakeholder groups can help improve understanding of MHPSS ethical programming standards and the importance of protecting them.
3. There are many different types of MHPSS services and support programs available to meet different needs of different populations in different contexts. HEART is one program, and although it has been used with great success in many locations, it is not the right fit for every context. In locations where the necessary conditions for successful HEART programming cannot be met, other approaches that are appropriate for local conditions can and should be used.

The fourth global challenge is staff turnover. Although staff turnover can be expected in every sector and in every location, it is particularly high in the global development and humanitarian response sectors. The sustainability of quality HEART programming relies on quality staffing. It is important to plan for a certain degree of staff turnover and equally important to invest in staff well-being to promote a positive work environment that supports staff retention. A few lessons learned related to this challenge include:

1. Provide multiple opportunities for staff development and recognition.
2. Ensure that training, mentoring, and monitoring of HEART is supportive and empowering for facilitators (as well as trainers, mentors, and monitors).
3. Encourage and support open communication amongst all stakeholders so that challenges can be solved in a supportive and collaborative way and successes can be celebrated collectively.

The challenges experienced by HEART are also applicable to other MHPSS services and programs, which leads us to our last reflection on lessons learned, which is the strength of community. Many of the challenges experienced in HEART have been overcome due to the support of a community of MHPSS colleagues across the global development and humanitarian response sectors. For HEART, these vital resources for problem solving and advocacy have helped the program to develop, adapt, and grow while maintaining ethical programming standards that ensure quality, fidelity, and sustainability. The final lesson learned related to global challenges is simply the importance of prioritizing communication and collaboration amongst a diverse set of global MHPSS professionals including those who work in health, education, and social support programming to collectively promote multi-layered and multi-sectoral MHPSS of which HEART is one part of a broad and holistic approach.

Lessons Learned through Key Points of Success

There are so many important components to the success of HEART in different settings, contexts, and locations around the world. Taking the time to adapt the global program model to the local setting before piloting is an important first step. Using a step-by-step approach to pilot the program followed by a period of review and revision before standardization and expansion in the local setting is also critical. Local partnerships, and coordination between partners, is a central component to quality scaling and sustainability. Maintaining ethical programming standards throughout every step of the process ensures quality and fidelity.

There are many more important lessons learned related to key points of HEART success, but we would like to specifically focus on the importance of HEART Champions, because every component that has contributed to the success of HEART has been possible because of champions who advocate for HEART at all levels of local and global operations across all relevant stakeholder groups. These champions are the greatest lesson learned from HEART success.

Within Save the Children, HEART Champions can be found in every office and department. They include global-, regional-, and country-based MHPSS professionals who provide direct support to local partners and practitioners, monitor program quality, manage program portfolios, support research, and organize advocacy activities. They also include fundraising staff, financial management staff, and office managers. Champions can be found everywhere, and their collective support creates a community of advocates within Save the Children that promote HEART, enabling it to continue to grow and expand with quality, fidelity, and sustainability.

HEART Champions can also be found outside of Save the Children, especially within local stakeholder groups including individuals within government agencies, national associations, local organizations, schools, and communities (including parents and children). Champions also exist within local donor groups where they advocate for funding to support scaling or sustaining HEART once scaling is complete. All these champions are critical to the success of HEART.

As we reflect on the role of HEART Champions, and everything that has contributed to the success of HEART, the most significant component of the program's success to date has been the sustainable funding commitments of key donors, including those who provide seed funding, scaling funding, and sustainability funding.

Spotlight on HEART Donor Champions

Of all the elements that have led to HEART's success, the greatest single contributing factor has been sustainable funding that provided the time needed to design the program, pilot, review, revise, standardize, expand, and adjust over time to meet new challenges in different local settings. Donor champions exist at the global, regional, and local level and play vital roles at different stages of HEART including the provision of Seed Funding, Scaling Funding, and Sustainability Funding. Seed funding from global donors provided for the original development of the global HEART program itself, and for launching the program in specific countries and locations around the world. Scaling funding from both global and local donors has allowed successful local HEART models to scale in specific locations. Sustainability funding from local donors has ensured that once scaling is complete, quality HEART programming will be able to continue to serve the children and communities it supports.

Seed Funding for the development of the global HEART program itself, and for launching the program in specific countries and locations.
Scaling Funding of local or country specific HEART programs once the local HEART model is ready to expand.
Sustainability Funding once HEART scaling has completed in a specific location.

The experience of one HEART donor champion provides important insight into the success of the global program. The Charles Engelhard Foundation has provided consistent funding for HEART since the start of the program. This started with seed funding that allowed Save the Children the time to design, test, and revise the program design over several years, to get the program right. It then supported several countries to pilot a local adaptation, review, revise, and standardize the program in the local setting before scaling. This type of multi-year funding commitment has been a critical element of the success of HEART design and scaling globally and has enabled HEART to maintain its ethical programming standards to ensure quality, fidelity, and sustainability.

Many of the country specific HEART program examples highlighted in this book started with seed funding from The Charles Engelhard Foundation. That funding covered the core costs of adapting the program to the local setting, training facilitators, providing arts supplies to schools and centers, and delivering facilitator mentoring and program monitoring to ensure quality and fidelity in the first few years that HEART piloted in each location. It provided local stakeholders the time to get it right before any major expansion began, and once the local model was working well, other donors, both local and international, were able to fund the next stages of HEART scaling and sustainability.

Charlene Engelhard, Director at The Charles Engelhard Foundation, is a Global HEART Donor Champion. Her personal experience with the arts, mental health, and philanthropy, offers a unique insight into the important role that an individual donor champion can have.

In Her Own Words, An Interview with Charlene Engelhard

I've had a consistent process of using the arts my whole life. For me, I started at around age 14, using the arts to overcome stressful or traumatic experiences in my life to support my mental health and I have used this my whole life and still today. For me, it was mostly painting, and sculpture. I felt it was an incredibly powerful tool and could see how it could help many children.

A lot of kids can't speak, they can't talk about what they experienced, and through the arts they can express it. When I was young, I couldn't put words to it, but the arts allowed me to. And this is what happens with kids in this program. They are given an opportunity to create art and have fun with their friends and things just come out. For me, I worked out everything that way, through painting, because I didn't have to use words, I could use my arts. Not everyone has access to therapy or mental health support and the arts can be that for many children.

Save the Children was great at fundraising to add to my seed funding. I gave the first batch of funding to get it started and then Save the Children raised more and made great partnerships with governments and other stakeholders, to make it really work.

If you are in philanthropy and you have funding and great ideas, you need to find the right partners and ones you trust. You need a relationship with the people in the organization that is strong and trusting so that the people in the organization can tell you what they need. I know the people in the program, and I trust them, and that is important. I have a very personal connection to these programs, so I want to see them through.

As a donor, you have to be really passionate about the subject you are funding and believe in its ultimate success. Also, you need to be in for the long run. Becoming personally involved in these programs has been super important for me, it's a very healing thing for me to be personally involved. You need to have the passion, the time, and commit to the long haul. The rewards are, well, there is no greater reward than going to a site visit and knowing that something you contributed to or supported is bringing such joy.

Also, as a donor, you have to learn how to be flexible. You have to have a lot of patience and you have to be willing to learn and see how things might need to change, because things change over time and the context becomes more complex and new stressors develop. Things don't always go the way you want because situations are sometimes out of our control – and the program can't just be a circus drop when the tent comes into town for only a short time – it needs to stay long term and adapt and expand to go to new places, so you need to be in it for the long run.

(Save the Children, 2023b)

The role of global and local HEART donor champions, from seed funding to scaling funding to funding the sustainability of the program at scale, is a cornerstone of HEART program success. Funding in ways that can complement existing infrastructure, build on existing strengths, and enable collaboration amongst partners has been a key point of success within HEART and one that has enabled collaboration amongst other champions and stakeholder groups. This supportive funding approach leads us to our final set of lessons learned, based on the experience of sustainable funding and supportive collaborations amongst stakeholder groups and the champions within them:

1. Only initiate HEART in locations where multi-year funding is available to ensure time and space to adapt, pilot, review and adjust, to get the local program model right to ensure quality, fidelity, and sustainability.
2. Coordinate global and local partners, and champions within those partners, in ways that recognize and appreciate individual and group contributions to support a holistic model of collaboration for program success.
3. Document program challenges, successes, and lessons learned, and share them with stakeholders and champions. The more knowledge and experience we all have, the better our collaborative work to support the well-being, learning, and development of children around the world.

Looking to the Future

The future of HEART looks promising as scaling efforts progress in multiple countries, local partnerships continue to develop, and new locations plan to pilot the program for the first time. As HEART continues to expand, and to adjust and adapt to new global, regional, and local challenges, we seek to continue to document best practices, share key points of learning, and promote art-based psychosocial support whenever and wherever possible. This book is one part of our commitment to document lessons learned and best practices. It is also an important moment for us to reflect on the enormous amount of hard work and dedication that so many colleagues, stakeholders, and champions contributed to get HEART to where it is today. We thank you for your commitments, we honor your contributions, and we look forward to bringing art-based psychosocial support, with quality, fidelity, and sustainability, to more children, families, and communities in the future.

Conclusion

Experiences of HEART challenges and successes have produced key points of learning that serve to inform and guide HEART programming worldwide. When adhering to ethical standards that ensure high quality training, mentoring, monitoring, and supplies, arts-based psychosocial support can be an effective, low cost, and sustainable approach to providing psychosocial support to children, families, and communities affected by adversity. We hope that the experience of HEART can serve to inform and promote arts-based psychosocial support approaches in more areas of global development, humanitarian response, and child support programming around the world.

Notes

1 Arts-based psychosocial support and its intended outcomes can be explained with diverse terminology including expressive arts, creative arts approaches, social emotional support, social emotional learning, social and emotional well-being, arts for well-being and development, and so on.
2 Inter-agency guidelines and resources from the Inter-Agency Standing Committee MHPSS Reference Group, WHO, IFRC, and others, can support strategies for maintaining ethical programming standards for MHPSS.

References

Abujaber, N., Vallières, F., McBride, K. A., Sheaf, G., Blum, P. T., Wiedemann, N., & Travers, Á. (2022). Examining the evidence for best practice guidelines in supportive supervision of lay health care providers in humanitarian emergencies: A systematic scoping review. *Journal of Global Health, 12*, 04017. https://doi.org/10.7189/jogh.12.04017

Ager, A., Pasha, E., Yu, G., Duke, T., Eriksson, C., & Cardozo, B. L. (2012). Stress, mental health, and burnout in national humanitarian aid workers in Gulu, Northern Uganda. *Journal of Traumatic Stress, 25*(6), 713–720. https://doi.org/10.1002/jts.21764

Ainsworth, M. D. S., Blehar, M. C., Waters, E., & Wall, S. (1978). *Patterns of attachment.* Erlbaum.

Aithal, S., Karkou, V., & Kuppusamy, G. (2020). Resilience enhancement in parents of children with an autism spectrum disorder through dance movement psychotherapy. *The Arts in Psychotherapy, 71*, 101–708. https://doi.org/10.1016/j.aip.2020.101708

Alodat, A. M., Alshagran, H. I., & Al-Bakkar, A. M. M. (2021). Psychosocial support services provided for Syrian refugees with disabilities: A systematic review and thematic analysis. *Middle East Current Psychiatry, 28*(1), 1–11. https://doi.org/10.1186/s43045-021-00144-2

American Academy of Pediatrics. (2012, April 29). *Being left out puts youths with special needs at risk for depression.* www.sciencedaily.com/releases/2012/04/120429085404.htm

Anda, R. F., Butchart, A., Felitti, V. J., & Brown, D. W. (2010). Building a framework for global surveillance of the public health implications of adverse childhood experiences. *American Journal of Preventive Medicine, 39*(1), 93–98. https://doi.org/10.1016/j.amepre.2010.03.015

Andersen S. L., Tomada, A., Vincow, E. S., Valente, E., Polcari, A., & Teicher, M. H. (2008). Preliminary evidence for sensitive periods in the effect of childhood sexual abuse on regional brain development. *Journal of Neuropsychiatry and Clinical Neuroscience, 20*(3), 292–301. https://doi.org/10.1176/jnp.2008.20.3.292

Arslanbek, A., Malhotra, B., & Kaimal, G. (2022). Indigenous and traditional arts in art therapy: Value, meaning, and clinical implications. *The Arts in Psychotherapy, 77*, 101879. https://doi.org/10.1016/j.aip.2021.101879

Asmussen, K., Fischer, F., Drayton, E., & McBride, T. (2020). *Adverse childhood experiences: what we know, what we don't know, and what should happen next.* Early

Intervention   Foundation.   www.eif.org.uk/report/adverse-childhood-experiences-what-we-know-what-we-dont-know-and-what-should-happen-next

Axline, V. M. (1969). *Play therapy* (Vol. 125). Ballantine Books.

Bardach, L., Yanagida, T., Gradinger, P., & Strohmeier, D. (2022). Understanding for which students and classes a socio-ecological aggression prevention program works best: Testing individual student and class level moderators. *Journal of Youth and Adolescence.* https://doi.org/ 10.1007/s10964-021-01553-6

Bardot, H. (2018). Art therapy training for relief workers to provide support and sustainability. *Journal of Applied Arts & Health, 9*(2), 157–169. https://doi.org/10.1386/jaah.9.2.157_1

Barnett, W. S. (1985). Benefit-cost analysis of the Perry Preschool Program and its policy implications. *Educational Evaluation and Policy Analysis, 7*(4), 333–342. https://doi.org/10.2307/1163569

Bartolomei, L., Eckert, R., & Pittaway, E. (2013). What happens there ... follows us here: Resettled but still at risk: Refugee women and girls in Australia. *Refuge, 30*(2), 45. https://doi.org/10.25071/1920-7336.39618

Basta, T. B., Shacham, E., & Reece, M. (2009). Symptoms of psychological distress: A comparison of rural and urban individuals enrolled in HIV-related mental health care. *AIDS Patient Care and STDs, 23*(12), 1053–1057. https://doi.org/10.1089/apc.2009.0193

Bearss, K. A., & DeSouza, J. F. X. (2021). Parkinson's disease motor symptom progression slowed with multisensory dance learning over 3-years: A preliminary longitudinal investigation. *Brain Sciences, 11*(7), 895. https://doi.org/ 10.3390/brainsci11070895

Bell, H., Shanti, K., & Dalton, L. (2003). Organizational prevention of vicarious trauma. *Families in Society, 84*(4), 463–470. https://doi.org/10.1606/1044-3894.131

Berberian, M. (2019). School-based art therapy: Filling the void. In M. Berberian & B. Davis (Eds.), *Art therapy practices for resilient youth: A strengths-based approach to at-promise children and adolescents* (pp. 425–446). Routledge.

Berenzon, S., Lara, M. A., & Medina-Mora, M. E. (2009). Inequity and poverty: everyday emotional disturbances and mental disorders in the Mexican urban population. *International Psychiatry, 6*(2), 32–34.

Berk, L. E. (2019). *Exploring child development*. Pearson.

Betancourt, T. S., Meyers-Ohki, S. E., Charrow, A., & Hansen, N. (2013). Annual research review: Mental health and resilience in HIV/AIDS-affected children–a review of the literature and recommendations for future research. *Journal of Child Psychology and Psychiatry, 54*(4), 423–444. https://doi.org/10.1111/j.1469-7610.2012.02613.x

Bettelheim, B. (1975/1976). *The uses of enchantment.* Vintage Books.

Bodrova, E. (2008). Make-believe play versus academic skills: a Vygotskian approach to today's dilemma of early childhood education. *European Early Childhood Education Research Journal, 16*(3), 357–369.

Bowlby, J. (1980). *Attachment and loss.* Basic Books.

Branson, D. C. (2019). Vicarious trauma, themes in research, and terminology: A review of literature. *Traumatology, 25*(1), 2–10. doi:10.1037/trm0000161

Briggs, C. A., & Bruscia, K. (1985). Developmental models for understanding musical behavior [Paper presentation]. Joint Conference on the Creative Arts Therapies, National Coalition of Arts Therapy Associations, New York

Briggs, C. (1991). A model for understanding musical development. *Music Therapy, 10*(1), 1–21. https://doi.org/10.1093/mt/10.1.1

Bronfenbrenner, U. (1979). *The ecology of human development: Experiments by nature and design*. Harvard University Press.

Bronfenbrenner, U. (Ed.). (2005). *Making human beings human*. Sage.

Brown, D., Hawkins-Rodgers, Y., & Kapadia, K. (2008). Multicultural considerations for the application of attachment theory. *American Journal of Psychotherapy, 62*(4), 353–363. https://doi.org/10.1176/appi.psychotherapy.2008.62.4.353

Brown, E. D., Garnett, M. L., Anderson, K. E., & Laurenceau, J. P. (2017). Can the arts get under the skin? Arts and cortisol for economically disadvantaged children. *Child Development, 88*(4), 1368–1381. https://doi.org/10.1111/cdev.12652

Brown, E. D., & Sax, K. L. (2013). Arts enrichment and preschool emotions for low-income children at risk. *Early Childhood Research Quarterly, 28*(2), 337–346. https://doi.org/10.1016/j.ecresq.2012.08.002

Bruscia, K. (1991). Musical origins: Developmental foundations for therapy. *Proceedings of the 18th Annual Conference of the Canadian Association for Music Therapy*, 210.

Campbell, P. S., & Scott-Kasner, C. (2019). *Music in childhood: From preschool through the elementary grades*. Cengage.

Caron, E., Bernard, K., & Metz, A. (2021). Fidelity and properties of the situation: Challenges and recommendations. In J. A. List, D. Suskind & L. H. Supplee (Eds.), *The scale-up effect in early childhood and public policy: Why interventions lose impact at scale and what we can do about it* (pp. 160–183). Routledge.

Carter, S., Dhaliwal, I., Friedlander, S., & Walsh, C. (2021). Forging collaborations for scale: Catalyzing partnerships among policy makers, practitioners, researchers, funders, and evidence-to-policy organizations. In J. A. List, D. Suskind & L. H. Supplee (Eds.), *The Scale-up effect in early childhood and public policy: Why interventions lose impact at scale and what we can do about it* (pp. 370–388). Routledge.

Centers for Disease Control and Prevention. (March 8, 2023a). *Mental health of children and parents-a strong connection*. www.cdc.gov/childrensmentalhealth/features/mental-health-children-and-parents.html#:~:text=The%20mental%20health%20of%20children,support%20their%20children's%20mental%20health.

Centers for Disease Control and Prevention. (June 29, 2023b). *Fast facts: Preventing adverse childhood experiences*. www.cdc.gov/violenceprevention/aces/fastfact.html

Center on the Developing Child. (2023). *Toxic stress*. Harvard University. https://developingchild.harvard.edu/science/key-concepts/toxic-stress/

Ćerimović, E. (2023). At risk and overlooked: Children with disabilities and armed conflict. *International Review of the Red Cross, 105*(922), 192–216. https://doi.org/10.1017/S181638312200087X

Champagne, E. R. & MacDonald, S. E. (2022). The perceived benefits of dance movement therapy for parents of a child on the autism spectrum: A pilot study. *The Arts in Psychotherapy, 77*, 101875. https://doi.org/10.1016/j.aip.2021.101875

Chemali, Z., Borba, C. P., Johnson, K., Hock, R. S., Parnarouskis, L., Henderson, D. C., & Fricchione, G. L. (2017). Humanitarian space and well-being: Effectiveness of training on a psychosocial intervention for host community-refugee interaction. *Medicine, Conflict and Survival, 33*(2), 141–161. https://doi.org/10.1080/13623699.2017.1323303

Chilcote, R. L. (2007). Art therapy with child tsunami survivors in Sri Lanka. *Art Therapy, 24*(4), 156–162. https://doi.org/10.1080/07421656.2007.10129475

Chilisa, B. (2012). *Indigenous research methodologies.* Sage.

Churiyah, M., Sholikhan, S., Filianti, F., & Sakdiyyah, D. A. (2020). Indonesia education readiness conducting distance learning in Covid-19 pandemic situation. *International Journal of Multicultural and Multireligious Understanding, 7*(6), 491–507. http://dx.doi.org/10.18415/ijmmu.v7i6.1833

Cocker, F., & Joss, N. (2016). Compassion fatigue among healthcare, emergency and community service workers: A systematic review. *International Journal of Environmental Research and Public Health, 13*(6), 618. https://doi.org/10.3390/ijerph13060618

Cohen, B. B. (2012). *Sensing, feeling, and action: The experiential anatomy of body-mind centering.* Wesleyan University Press.

Cohen-Katz, J., Wiley, S. D., Capuano, T., Baker, D. M., & Shapiro, S. (2005). The effects of mindfulness-based stress reduction on nurse stress and burnout, Part II: A quantitative and qualitative study. *Holistic Nursing Practice, 19*(1), 26–35. https://doi.org/10.1097/00004650-200501000-00008

Cohen, S., Kamarck, T., & Mermelstein, R. (1983). A global measure of perceived stress. *Journal of Health and Social Behavior, 24*(4), 385–396. https://doi.org/10.2307/2136404

Collier, A. F. (2011). The well-being of women who create with textiles: Implications for art therapy. *Art Therapy, 28*(3), 104–112. https://doi.org/10.1080/07421656.2011.597025

Collier, A.F. (2012). *Using textile arts and handcrafts in therapy with women.* Jessica Kingsley.

Compas, B. E., Orosan, P. G., & Grant, K. E. (1993). Adolescent stress and coping: Implications for psychopathology during adolescence. *Journal of Adolescence, 16*(3), 331–349. https://doi.org/10.1006/jado.1993.1028

Compas, B. E., & Wagner, B. M. (2017). Psychosocial stress during adolescence: Intrapersonal and interpersonal processes. In M. E. Colten & S. Gore (Eds.) *Adolescent stress: Causes and Consequences* (pp. 67–86). Routledge.

Conference of State Parties to the Convention on the Rights of Persons with Disabilities. (2021). *Protecting the Rights of Persons with Disabilities in Armed Conflict and Humanitarian Emergencies.* https://documents-dds-ny.un.org/doc/UNDOC/GEN/N21/078/66/PDF/N2107866.pdf?OpenElement

Core Humanitarian Standard (CHS) Alliance, ICVA Network (2021). *Leading well: Aid leader perspectives on staff well-being and organizational culture.* https://d1h79zlghft2zs.cloudfront.net/uploads/2021/04/Leading-well-report-CHS-Alliance.pdf

Crain, W. (2015). *Theories of development: Concepts and applications* (8th Ed). Routledge.

Crampin, A. C., Floyd, S., Fine, P. E. M., Glynn, J. R., Madise, N., Nyondo, A., Khondowe, M. M., Njoka, C. L., Kanyongoloka, H., Ngwira, B., & Zaba, B. (2003). The long-term impact of HIV and orphanhood on the mortality and physical well-being of children in rural Malawi. *AIDS, 17*(3), 389–397. https://doi.org/10/1097/00002030-200302140-00013

Crawford, M. (2020). Ecological systems theory: Exploring the development of the theoretical framework as conceived by Bronfenbrenner. *Journal of Public Health Issues and Practices*, *4*(2), 170. https://doi.org/10.33790/jphip1100170

Csikszentmihalyi, M. (2013). *Creativity: The psychology of discovery and invention*. Harper Perennial Modern Classics.

Cucca, A., Acosta, I., Berberian, M., Lemen, A. C., Rizzo, J. R., Ghilardi, M. F., Quartarone, A., Feigin, A. S., Di Rocco, A., & Biagioni, M. C. (2018). Visuospatial exploration and art therapy intervention in patients with Parkinson's disease: An exploratory therapeutic protocol. *Complementary Therapies in Medicine*, *40*, 70–76. https://doi.org/10.1016/j.ctim.2018.07.011

Darney, D., Reinke, W. M., Herman, K. C., Stormont, M., & Ialongo, N. S. (2013). Children with co-occurring academic and behaviour problems in first grade: Distal outcomes in twelfth grade. *Journal of School Psychology*, *51*(1), 117–128. https://doi.org/10.1016/j.jsp.2012.09.005

Davies, D. (2010). Enhancing the role of the arts in primary pre-service teacher education. *Teaching and Teacher Education*, *26*(3), 630–638. https://doi.org/10.1016/j.tate.2009.09.011

Davies, C., Knuiman, M., & Rosenberg, M. (2016). The art of being mentally healthy: A study to quantify the relationship between recreational arts engagement and mental well-being in the general population. *BMC Public Health*, 16, 15.

Desautels, L. (2020). *Connections over compliance: Rewiring our perceptions of discipline*. Wyatt-MacKenzie Publishing.

Desautels, L. (2021). *Sensory and nervous system practices*. Revelationsineducation.com.

Dettweiler, U., Becker, C., Auestad, B. H., Simon, P., & Kirsch, P. (2017). Stress in school: Some empirical hints on the circadian cortisol rhythm of children in outdoor and indoor classes. *International Journal of Environmental Research and Public Health*, *14*(5), 475. https://doi.org/10.3390/ijerph14050475

Diamond, K. E., Hong, S. Y., & Tu, H. (2008). Context influences preschool children's decisions to include a peer with a physical disability in play. *Exceptionality*, *16*(3), 141–155. https://doi.org/10.1080/09362830802198328

Dikyurt, A. E. (2023). Bosnian Americans: Transmission of trauma between generations. *Journal of Aggression, Conflict and Peace Research*, *15*(4), 301–311. https://doi.org/10.1108/JACPR-08-2022-0736

Dix, K., Shearer, J., Slee, P., & Butcher, C. (2010). *KidsMatter for students with a disability: Evaluation report*. Ministerial Advisory Committee: Students with Disabilities. https://www.researchgate.net/publication/280094099_KidsMatter_for_Students_with_a_Disability_Evaluation_Report.

Doom, J. R., Seok, D., Narayan, A. J., & Fox, K. R. (2021). Adverse and benevolent childhood experiences predict mental health during the COVID-19 pandemic. *Adversity and Resilience Science*, *2*(3), 1–12. https://doi.org/10.1007/s42844-021-00038-6

Dubow, E. F., Boxer, P., Huesmann, L. R., Landau, S., Dvir, S., Shikaki, K., & Ginges, J. (2012). Cumulative effects of exposure to violence on posttraumatic stress in Palestinian and Israeli youth. *Journal of Clinical Child and Adolescent Psychology*, *41*(6), 837–844. https://doi.org/10.1080/15374416.2012.675571

Dunn, E. C., Solovieff, N., Lowe, S. R., Gallagher, P. J., Chaponis, J., Rosand, J., Koenen, K. C., Waters, M. C., Rhodes, J. E., & Smoller, J. W. (2014). Interaction between genetic variants and exposure to Hurricane Katrina on post-traumatic stress and post-traumatic growth: A prospective analysis of low income adults. *Journal of Affective Disorders, 152–154*(2014), 243–249. https://doi.org/10.1016/j.jad.2013.09.018

Dutton, D. (2010). *The art instinct: Beauty, pleasure and human evolution.* Bloomsbury Press.

Edwards, B. M., Smart, E., King, G., Curran, C. J., & Kingsnorth, S. (2020). Performance and visual arts-based programs for children with disabilities: A scoping review focusing on psychosocial outcomes. *Disability and Rehabilitation, 42*(4), 574–585. https://doi.org/10.1080/09638288.2018.1593734

Epp, K. M. (2008). Outcome-based evaluation of a social skills program using art therapy and group therapy for children on the autism spectrum. *Children & Schools, 30*(1), 27–36. https://doi.org/10.1093/cs/30.1.27

Erikson, E. H. (1950). *Childhood and society.* W. W. Norton & Company, Inc.

Eriksson, C. B., Bjorck, J. P., Larson, L. C., Walling, S. M., Trice, G. A., Fawcett, J., Abernethy, A. D., & Foy, D. W. (2009). Social support, organizational support, and religious support in relation to burnout in expatriate humanitarian aid workers. *Mental Health, Religion and Culture, 12*(7), 671–686. https://doi.org/10.1080/13674670903029146

Ernst, M., Niederer, D., Werner, A. M., Czaja, S. J., Mikton, C., Ong, A. D., Rosen, T., Brähler, E., & Beutel, M. E. (2022). Loneliness before and during the COVID-19 pandemic: A systematic review with meta-analysis. *The American Psychologist, 77*(5), 660–677. https://doi.org/10.1037/amp0001005

European Civil Protection and Humanitarian Aid Operations. (2023). *Uganda factsheet.* European Commission. https://civil-protection-humanitarian-aid.ec.europa.eu/where/africa/uganda_en#what-are-the-needs

European Commission (2023). *European Civil Protection and Humanitarian Aid Operations: Uganda.* https://civil-protection-humanitarian-aid.ec.europa.eu/where/africa/uganda_en#what-are-the-needs

Fancourt, D., & Finn, S. (2019). What is the evidence on the role of the arts in improving health and well-being? A scoping review. WHO Regional Office for Europe. https://apps.who.int/iris/handle/10665/329834

Ferguson, K. T., Cassells, R. C., MacAllister, J. W., & Evans, G. W. (2013). The physical environment and child development: An international review. *International Journal of Psychology, 48*(4), 437–468. https://doi.org/ 10.1080/00207594.2013.804190

Fields, L., & Prinz, R. J. (1997). Coping and adjustment during childhood and adolescence. *Clinical Psychology Review, 17*(8), 937–976. https://doi.org/10.1016/S0272-7358(97)00033-0

Figley, C. R. (1995). *Compassion fatigue: Coping with secondary traumatic stress disorder in those who treat the traumatized.* Brunner-Routledge.

Figley, C. R. (1999). Compassion fatigue: Toward a new understanding of the costs of caring. In B. H. Stamm (Ed.), *Secondary Traumatic Stress: Self-care Issues for Clinicians, Researchers, & Educators* (2nd ed., pp. 3–28). Sidran Press.

Figley, C. R. (Ed.). (2002). *Treating compassion fatigue.* Brunner-Routledge.

Fischer, K. W., & Bidell, T. R. (2006). Dynamic development of action and thought. In R. M. Lerner & W. Damon (Eds.), *Handbook of child psychology: Theoretical models of human development* (6th ed., pp. 313–399). John Wiley & Sons, Inc.

Flinn, M. V., & England, B. G. (1995). Childhood stress and family environment. *CurrentAnthropology , 36*(5), 854–866. https://doi.org/10.1086/204444

Frank, S. M., Becker, M., Qi, A., Geiger, P., Frank, U. I., Rosedahl, L. A., Malloni, W. M., Sasaki, Y., Greenlee, M. W., & Watanabe, T. (2022). Efficient learning in children with rapid GABA boosting during and after training. *Current Biology*, *32*(23), 5022–5030. e7. https://doi.org/10.1016/j.cub.2022.10.021

Franke, H. A. (2014). Toxic stress: effects, prevention and treatment. *Children*, *1*(3), 390–402. https://doi.org/10.3390/children1030390

Frankish, P. (2018). *Disability psychotherapy: An innovative approach to trauma-informed care* (1st ed.). Routledge.

Frankl, V. (1946). *Man's search for meaning.* Beacon Press

Franklin, M. F. (2018). *Art as contemplative practice: Expressive pathways to the self.* SUNY Press.

Freilich, R., & Shechtman, Z. (2010). The contribution of art therapy to the social, emotional, and academic adjustment of children with learning disabilities. *The Arts in Psychotherapy*, *37*(2), 97–105. https://doi.org/ 10.1016/j.aip.2010.02.003

Friedlander, S., & Perks, B. (2022). *Caregiver mental health and well-being: The key to thriving families. Supporting children means supporting caregivers too.* United Nations Children's Fund. www.unicef.org/blog/caregiver-mental-health-well-being-key-thriving-families

Friston K., & Kiebel, S. (2009). Predictive coding under the free-energy principle. *Philosophical Translation of the Royal Society B: Biological Sciences*, 12, *364*(1521), 1211–1221. https:doi.org// 10.1098/rstb.2008.0300. PMID: 19528002; PMCID: PMC2666703.

Furlager, A. (2018). Training of trainers: Psychosocial training for teachers for a safe educational environment. *Journal of Applied Arts & Health*, *9*(2), 213–221. https:// doi.org/ 10.1386/jaah.9.2.213_1

Gabriels, R. L. (2003). Art therapy with children who have autism and their families. In C. A. Malchiodi (Ed.), *Handbook of Art Therapy* (pp.193–206). Guilford Press.

Garrison, K., Caiola, N., Sullivan, R., & Lynam, P. (2004). *Supervising Healthcare Services: Improving the Performance of People.* JHPIEGO. https://pdf.usaid.gov/pdf_docs/PNACX168.pdf

Gavron, T., Eskenasy, N., Snir, S., Bat-Or, M., Fernandez, K. G., & Ocampo, M. T. W. (2022). Arts-based psychosocial training after the Yolanda typhoon in the Philippines. *The Arts in Psychotherapy*, *80*, 101936. https://doi.org/10.1016/j.aip.2022.101936

Gavron, T., & Shemesh, H. (2022). "I am actually growing my art": Building an expressive terrarium as an intervention tool in arts therapy. *Journal of Creativity in Mental Health*, *19*(1), 24–38. https://doi.org/10.1080/15401383.2022.2119184

Gentry, J. E., Baranowsky, A. B., & Dunning, K. (2002). ARP: The accelerated recovery program (ARP) for compassion fatigue. In C. R. Figley (Ed.), *Treating Compassion Fatigue* (pp. 123–137). Brunner-Routledge.

Gibson, M. A., & Larson, M. A. (2007). Visual arts and academic achievement. *Journal for Learning through the Arts*, *3*(1), 8. https://doi.org/10.21977/D93110057

Gilman, L. (2011). *The dance of politics: Gender, performance, and democratization in Malawi* (Vol. 9). Temple University Press.

Gilman, L. (2015). Demonic or cultural treasure? Local perspectives on Vimbuza, intangible cultural heritage, and UNESCO in Malawi. *Journal of Folklore Research*, *52*(2–3), 199–216. https://doi.org/10.2979/jfolkrese.52.2-3.199

Goodman, G., Dent, V. F., Tuman, D., & Lee, S. (2022). Drawings from a play-based intervention: Windows to the soul of rural Ugandan preschool children's artistic development. *The Arts in Psychotherapy, 77*, 1–10. https://doi.org/10.1016/j.aip.2021.101876

Gordon, E. E. (2012). *Learning sequences in music: A contemporary music learning theory.* GIA Publications.

Goswami, U. (2008). *Cognitive development: The learning brain.* Routledge.

Gottfried, T., Elefant, C., & Gold, C. (2022). Music-oriented parent counseling to promote improvement in level of parental stress, quality of life and the use of music in everyday life among parents of children with autism: A mixed-methods randomized controlled study. *Nordic Journal of Music Therapy*, 1–26. https://doi.org/10.1080/08098131.2022.2131890

Greenberg, M. T., Cicchetti, D., & Cummings, E. M. (Eds.) (1990). *Attachment in the preschool years: Theory, research, and intervention.* University of Chicago Press.

Gupta, A., & Singhal, N. (2005). Psychosocial support for families of children with autism. *Asia Pacific Disability Rehabilitation Journal, 16*(2), 62–83.

Gupta, S., Supplee, L.H., Suskind, D., & List, J.A., (2021). Failed to scale: embracing the challenge of scaling in early childhood. In J. A. List, D. Suskind & L. H. Supplee (Eds.), *The scale-up effect in early childhood and public policy: Why interventions lose impact at scale and what we can do about it* (pp. 1–21). Routledge.

Guzzino, M., & Taxis, C. (1995). Leading experiential vicarious trauma groups for professionals. *Treating Abuse Today, 4*, 27–31.

Hackman, D. A., & Farah, M. J. (2009). Socioeconomic status and the developing brain. *Trends in Cognitive Sciences, 13*(2), 65–73. https://doi.org/10.1016/j.tics.2008.11.003

Hackney, P. (1998). *Making connections: Total body integration through Bartenieff fundamentals.* Gordon and Breach.

Haiblum-Itskovitch, S., Czamanski-Cohen, J., & Galili, G. (2018). Emotional response and changes in heart rate variability following art-making with three different art materials. *Front Psychol., 18*(9), 968. doi: 10.3389/fpsyg.2018.00968.

Hair, N. L. Hanson, J. L., Wolfe, B. L., & Pollak, S. D. (2015). Association of child poverty, brain development, and academic achievement. *JAMA Pediatrics, 169*(9), 822–829. https://doi.org/10.1001 /jamapediatrics.2015.1475.

Hannan, S. A. (2022). *Fostering inclusion in Mexico.* International Monetary Fund. www.imf.org/en/News/Articles/2022/01/24/cf-fostering-inclusion-in-mexico

Hardiman, M., Rinne, L., & Yarmolinskaya, J. (2014). The effects of arts integration on long term retention of academic content. *Mind, Brain and Education, 8*(3), 144–148. https://doi.org/10.1111/mbe.12053

Hastings, R. P., & Johnson, E. (2001). Stress in UK families conducting intensive home-based behavioral intervention for their young child with autism. *Journal of Autism and Developmental Disorders, 31*(3), 327–336. https://doi.org/10.1023/A:1010799329795

Hays-Grudo, J., & Morris, A. S. (2020). *Adverse and protective childhood experiences: A developmental perspective.* American Psychological Association.

Heckman, J. J. (2006). Skill formation and the economics of investing in disadvantaged children. *Science, 312*(5782),1900–1902. https://doi.org/10.1126/science.1128898

Heim, C. M., Mayberg, H. S., Mletzko, T., Nemeroff, C. B., & Pruessner, J. C. (2013). Decreased cortical representation of genital somatosensory field after childhood sexual abuse. *The American Journal of Psychiatry*, *170*(6), 616–623. https://doi.org/10.1176/appi.ajp.2013.12070950

Heiman, T. (2021). Parents' voice: Parents' emotional and practical coping with a child with special needs. *Psychology*, *12*(5), 675–691. https://doi.org/10.4236/psych.2021.125042

Hepsomali, P., Machon, S., Barker, H., Lythgoe, D. J., Hugdahl, K., Gudbrandsen, M., & Allen, P. (2023). Signatures of exposure to childhood trauma in young adults in the structure and neurochemistry of the superior temporal gyrus. *Journal of Psychopharmacology*, *37*(5), 510–519. https://doi.org/10.1177/02698811231168243

Hernández, P., Gangsei, D., & Engstrom, D. (2007). Vicarious resilience: A new concept in work with those who survive trauma. *Family Process*, *46*(2), 229–241. https://doi.org/10.1111/j.1545-5300.2007.00206.x

Hernandez-Wolfe, P. (2018). Vicarious resilience: A comprehensive review. *Revista de Estudios Sociales*, *66*, 9–17. https://doi.org/10.7440/res66.2018.02

Herzog, J. I., & Schmahl, C. (2018). Adverse childhood experiences and the consequences on neurobiological, psychosocial, and somatic conditions across the lifespan. *Frontiers in Psychiatry*, *9*, 420. https://doi.org/10.3389/fpsyt.2018.00420

Hinz, L. D. (2009). *Expressive therapies continuum: A framework for using art in therapy*. Routledge.

Hirsh-Pasek, K., Golinkoff, R. M., Berk, L. E., & Singer, D. G. (2009). *A mandate for playful learning in preschool: Presenting the evidence*. Oxford University Press.

Ho, L. L. K., Li, W. H. C., Cheung, A. T., Luo, Y., Xia, W., & Chung, J. O. K. (2022). Impact of poverty on parent–child relationships, parental stress, and parenting practices. *Frontiers in Public Health*, *10*, 849408. https://doi.org/10.3389/fpubh.2022.849408

Holz, N. E., Zabihi, M., Kia, S. M., Monninger, M., Aggensteiner, P., Siehl, S., Floris, D. L., Bokde, A. L. W., Desrivières, S., Flor, H., Grigis, A., Garavan, H., Gowland, P., Heinz, A., Brühl, R., Martinot, J., Martinot, M. P., Orfanos, D. P., Paus, T. … Marquand, A. F. (2023). A stable and replicable neural signature of lifespan adversity in the adult brain. *Nature Neuroscience*, *26*(9), 1603–1612. https://doi.org/10.1038/s41593-023-01410-8

Holtz, C. A., Fox, R. A., & Meurer, J. R. (2015). Incidence of behavior problems in toddlers and preschool children from families living in poverty. *Journal of Psychology*, *149*(2), 161–74. https://doi.org/10.1080/00223980.2013.853020

Horwitz, M. (1998). Social worker trauma: Building resilience in child protection social workers. *Smith College Studies in Social Work*, *68*(3), 363–377. https://doi.org/10.1080/00377319809517536

Hoshino, J., & Cameron, C. (2008). Narrative art therapy within a multicultural framework, in C. Kerr & J. Hoshino (Eds.), *Family Art Therapy: Foundations of Theory and Practice* (pp. 193–219). Routledge.

Hsiao, Y. J. (2018). Parental stress in families of children with disabilities. *Intervention in School and Clinic*, *53*(4), 201–205. https://doi.org/10.1177/1053451217712956

Huss, E., Kaufman, R., Avgar, A., & Shuker, E. (2016). Arts as a vehicle for community building and post-disaster development. *Disasters*, *40*(2), 284–303. https://doi.org/10.1111/disa.12143

Huss, E., Sarid, O., & Cwikel, J. (2010). Using art as a self-regulating tool in a war situation: A model for social workers. *Health & Social Work, 35*(3), 201–209. https://doi.org/10.1093/hsw/35.3.201

Hussain, S. (2010). Art therapy for children who have survived disaster. *AMA Journal of Ethics, 12*(9), 750–753. https://doi.org/10.1001/virtualmentor.2010.12.9.imhl1-1009

Inter-Agency Standing Committee. (2007). *IASC guidelines on mental health and psychosocial support in emergency settings.* https://interagencystandingcommittee.org/iasc-task-force-mental-health-and-psychosocial-support-emergency-settings/iasc-guidelines-mental-health-and-psychosocial-support-emergency-settings-2007

Inter-Agency Standing Committee. (2020). *IASC guidance on basic psychosocial skills: A guide for COVID-19 responders.* https://interagencystandingcommittee.org/iasc-reference-group-mental-health-and-psychosocial-support-emergency-settings/iasc-guidance-basic-psychosocial-skills-guide-covid-19-responders

Inter-Agency Standing Committee. (2024, January 15). *IASC Information note on disability and inclusion in MHPSS.* https://interagencystandingcommittee.org/iasc-reference-group-mental-health-and-psychosocial-support-emergency-settings/iasc-information-note-disability-and-inclusion-mhpss

Inter-Agency Standing Committee (forthcoming). *Accessible consultation and meaningful participation of organisations of persons with disabilities (OPD).*

Ireland, M. J., Clough, B., Gill, K., Langan, F., O'Connor, A., & Spencer, L. (2017). A randomized controlled trial of mindfulness to reduce stress and burnout among intern medical practitioners. *Medical Teacher, 39*(4), 409–414. https://doi.org/10.1080/0142159X.2017.1294749

Izard, C. E., King, K. A., Trentacosta, C. J., Morgan, J. K., Laurenceau, J. P., Krauthamer-Ewing, E. S., & Finlon, K. J. (2008). Accelerating the development of emotion competence in Head Start children: Effects on adaptive and maladaptive behavior. *Development and Psychopathology, 20*(1), 369–397. https://doi.org/10.1017/S0954579408000175

Jachens, L. (2019). Humanitarian aid workers' mental health and duty of care. *Europe's Journal of Psychology, 15*(4), 650–655. https://doi.org/10.5964/ejop.v15i4.2221

Jarvis, J. M. (2011). Promoting mental health through inclusive pedagogy. In R. H. Shute, P. T. Slee, R. Murray-Harvey, & K. L. Dix (Eds.), *Mental health and wellbeing: Educational perspectives* (pp. 237–248). Shannon Research Press.

Jones, L., Bellis, M. A., Wood, S., Hughes, K., McCoy, E., Eckley, L., Bates, G., Mikton, C., Shakespeare, T., & Officer, A. (2012). Prevalence and risk of violence against children with disabilities: A systematic review and meta-analysis of observational studies. *The Lancet, 380*(9845), 899–907. https://doi.org/10.1016/S0140-6736(12)60692-8

Jordan, K., & Tseris, E. (2018). Locating, understanding and celebrating disability: Revisiting Erikson's "stages." *Feminism & Psychology, 28*(3), 427–444. https://doi.org/10.1177/0959353517705400

Kagitcibasi, C. (2007). *Family, self, and human development across cultures: Theory and applications.* Routledge.

Kaimal, G. (2022). *The expressive instinct: How imagination and creative works help us survive and thrive.* Oxford University Press.

Kaimal, G., & Arslanbek, A. (2020). Indigenous and traditional visual artistic practices: Implications for art therapy clinical practice and research. *Frontiers in Psychology*, *11*, 1320. https://doi.org/10.3389/fpsyg.2020.01320

Kaimal, G., Carroll-Haskins, K., Mensinger, J. L., Dieterich-Hartwell, R. M., Manders, E., & Levin, W. P. (2019). Outcomes of art therapy and coloring for professional and informal caregivers of patients in a radiation oncology unit: A mixed-methods pilot study. *European Journal of Oncology Nursing*, *42*, 153–161. https://doi.org/ 10.1016/ j.ejon.2019.08.006

Kaimal, G., Carroll-Haskins, K., Topoglu, Y., Ramakrishnan, A., Arslanbek, A., & Ayaz, H. (2021). Exploratory fNIRS assessment of differences in activation in virtual reality visual self-expression including with a fragrance stimulus. *Art Therapy*, *39*(3), 128–137.

Kaimal, G., Councill, T., Ramsey, K. Cottone, C. A., & Snyder, K. (2019). A conceptual framework for research in art therapy research in pediatric hematology and oncology settings. *Canadian Art Therapy Association Journal*, *32*(2), 95–103. https://doi.org/ 10.1080/08322473.2019.1672453.

Kaimal, G., Hommel, S., Seiden, J., & Pisani, L. (2022). Healing and Education Through the Arts (HEART): Outcomes of a 9-month arts-based psychosocial support intervention for 5-year-old children in Malawi. In C. Maguire and A. Holt (Eds.), *Arts and culture in global development practice: Expression, identity, and empowerment* (pp. 104–117). Routledge. https://doi.org/10.4324/9781003148203-7

Kaimal, G., Mensinger, J. L., & Carroll-Haskins, K., (2020). Outcomes of collage artbased and narrative self-expression among home hospice caregivers. *International Journal of Art Therapy*, *25*(2), 52–63. https://doi.org/10.1080/17454832.2020.1752756

Kaimal, G., Ray, K., & Muniz, J. (2016). Reduction of cortisol levels and participants' responses following art making. *Art Therapy*, *33*(2), 74–80. https://doi.org/10.1080/ 07421656.2016.1166832

Kaku, S. M., Sibeoni, J., Basheer, S., Chang, J. P. C., Dahanayake, D. M. A., Irarrazaval, M., Lachman, J. M., Mapayi, B. M., Mejia, A., Orri, M., Jui-Goh, T., Uddin, M. S., & Vallance, I. (2022). Global child and adolescent mental health perspectives: Bringing change locally, while thinking globally. *Child and Adolescent Psychiatry and Mental Health*, *16*(1), 1–82. https://doi.org/10.1186/s13034-022-00512-8

Kalmanowitz, D. (2016). Inhabited studio: Art therapy and mindfulness, resilience, adversity and refugees. *International Journal of Art Therapy*, *21*(2), 75–84. https:// doi.org/10.1080/17454832.2016.1170053

Kamali, M., Munyuzangabo, M., Siddiqui, F. J., Gaffey, M. F., Meteke, S., Als, D., Jain, R. P., Radhakrishnan, A., Shah, S., Ataullahjan, A., & Bhutta, Z. A. (2020). Delivering mental health and psychosocial support interventions to women and children in conflict settings: A systematic review. *BMJ Global Health*, *5*(3), e002014. https://doi.org/ 10.1136/bmjgh-2019-002014

Kandel, E. (2012). *The age of insight: The quest to understand the unconscious in mind, art and brain*. Random House.

Kapur, M. (2023, April 10). *Childcare in ancient India: A life span approach*. Indian Psychology Institute. https://ipi.org.in/texts/others/malvikakapur-childcare-sp.php

Kaufman, J. C., & Beghetto, R. A. (2009). Beyond big and little: The four c model of creativity. *Review of General Psychology*, *13*(1), 1–12. https://doi.org/10.1037/a0013688

Kellogg, R., & O'Dell, S. (1967) *The psychology of children's art*. CRM Incorporated.

Kerns, C. M., Newschaffer, C. J., & Berkowitz, S. J. (2015). Traumatic childhood events and autism spectrum disorder. *Journal of Autism and Developmental Disorders*, *45*(11), 3475–3486. https://doi.org/10.1007/s10803-015-2392-y

Kerns, C. M., Newschaffer, C. J., Berkowitz, S., & Lee, B. K. (2017). Brief report: Examining the association of autism and adverse childhood experiences in the national survey of children's health: The important role of income and co-occurring mental health conditions. *Journal of Autism and Developmental Disorders*, *47*(7), 2275–2281. https://doi.org/10.1007/s10803-017-3111-7

Kestenberg Amighi, J., Loman, S., & Sossin, K. M. (2018). *The meaning of movement:Embodied development, clinical and cultural perspectives of the Kestenberg Movement Profile* (2nd ed.). Routledge.

Klein, M. (1955). The psychoanalytic play technique. *American Journal of Orthopsychiatry*, *25*(2), 223–237. https://doi.org/10.1111/j.1929-0025.1955. tb00131.x

Kloep, M., Hendry, L. B., Taylor, R., & Stuart-Hamilton, I. (2016). *Development from adolescence to early adulthood: A dynamic systemic approach to transitions and transformations*. Psychology Press.

Klorer, P. G., & Robb, M. (2012). Art enrichment: Evaluating a collaboration between Headstart and a graduate art therapy program. *Art Therapy*, *24*(4),180–187. https://doi. org/10.1080/07421656.2012.730920

Knight, C. (2013). Indirect trauma: Implications for self-care, supervision, the organization, and the academic institution. *The Clinical Supervisor*, *32*(2), 224–243. https:// doi.org/10.1080/07325223.2013.850139

Kohrt, B. A., & Carruth, L. (2022). Syndemic effects in complex humanitarian emergencies: A framework for understanding political violence and improving multi-morbidity health outcomes. *Social Science & Medicine*, *295*, 113378. https://doi.org/10.1016/ j.socscimed.2020.113378

Kousky, C. (2016). Impacts of natural disasters on children. *The Future of Children*, *26*(1), 73–92. https://doi.org/10.1353/foc.2016.0004

Kovács, K. E., Dan, B., Hrabéczy, A., Bacskai, K., & Pusztai, G. (2022). Is resilience a trait or a result of parental involvement? The results of a systematic literature review. *Education Sciences*, *12*(6), 372. https://doi.org/10.3390/educsci12060372

Kozulin, A., & Gindis, B. (2007). Sociocultural theory and education of children with special needs: From defectology to remedial pedagogy. In H. Daniels, M. Cole, & J. V. Wertsch (Eds.), *The Cambridge companion to Vygotsky* (pp. 332–362). Cambridge University Press. https://doi.org/10.1017/CCOL0521831040.014

Kumru, A., Bugan, B., & Gülseven, Z. (2019). Parenting and prosocial moral behavior in predominantly Muslim countries. In D. J. Laible, G. Carlo, & L. M. Padilla-Walker (Eds.), *The Oxford handbook of parenting and moral development* (pp 227–246). Oxford University Press. https://doi.org/10.1093/oxfordhb/9780190638696.013.4

Lai, N. (2011). Expressive Arts Therapy for Mother–Child Relationship (EAT-MCR): A novel model for domestic violence survivors in Chinese culture. *The Arts in Psychotherapy*, *38*(5), 305–311. https://doi.org/10.1016/j.aip.2011.08.001

Lambert, K. (2008). *Lifting depression: A neuroscientist's hands-on approach to activating your brain's healing power*. Basic Books.

Landreth, G. L. (2012). *Play therapy: The art of the relationship.* Routledge.

Lata, S., & Verma, S. (2013). Mental health of HIV/AIDS orphans: A review. *Journal of AIDS and HIV Research, 5*(12), 455–467. https://doi.org/10.5897/JAHR2013.0271

Lazarus, R. S., & Folkman, S. (1984). *Stress, appraisal, and coping.* Springer Publishing.

Lerner, R. M. (Ed.), *Handbook of child psychology: Vol. 1. Theoretical Models of human development* (6th ed.). Wiley.

Levick, M. F. (1983). *They could not talk and so they drew: Children's styles of coping and thinking.* Charles C. Thomas Publishers.

Lévi-Strauss, C. (1950). *Structural anthropology.* Basic Books.

Limb, J., & Braun, A. R. (2008). Neural substrates of spontaneous musical performance: An fMRI Study of Jazz Improvisation. *PLoS ONE, 3*(2): e1679. https://doi.org/10.1371/journal.pone.0001679

Ling J., Zahry, N. R., & Liu, C. (2021). Stress management interventions among socioeconomically disadvantaged parents: A meta-analysis and moderation analysis. *International Journal of Nursing Studies, 120,* 103954. https://doi.org/10.1016/j.ijnurstu.2021.103954.

Linnan, L., Fisher, E. B., & Hood, S. (2013). The power and potential of peer support in workplace interventions. *American Journal of Health Promotion, 28*(1), TAHP2–TAH10. https://doi.org/10.4278/ajhp.120316-QUAN-143

Lobo, Y. B., & Winsler, A. (2006). The effects of a creative dance and movement program on the social competence of Head Start preschoolers. *Social Development, 15*(3), 501–519. https://doi.org/10.1111/j.1467-9507.2006.00353.x

Lopes-Cardozo, B., Gotway Crawford, C., Eriksson, C., Zhu, J., Sabin, M., Ager, A., Foy, D., Snider, L., Scholte, W., Kaiser, R., Olff, M., Rijnen, B., Simon, W., & Uddin, M. (2012). Psychological distress, depression, anxiety, and burnout among international humanitarian aid workers: A longitudinal study. *PLoS One, 7*(9), e44948. https://doi.org/10.1371/journal.pone.0044948

Lowenfeld, V., & Brittain, W. L. (1987). *Creative and mental growth* (8th ed.). Prentice-Hall Incorporated.

Luby, J., Belden, A., Botteron, K., Marrus, N., Harms, M. P., Babb, C., Tomoyuki, N., & Barch, D. (2013). The effects of poverty on childhood brain development: The mediating effect of caregiving and stressful life events. *JAMA Pediatrics, 167*(12), 1135–1142. https://doi.org/10.1001/jamapediatrics.2013.3139

Luby, S., Deneault, A., Racine, N., Park, J., Thiemann, R., Zhu, J., Dimitropoulos, G., Williamson, T., Fearon, P., Cénat, J. M., McDonald, S., Devereux, C., & Neville, R. D. (2023). Adverse childhood experiences: A meta-analysis of prevalence and moderators among half a million adults in 206 studies. *World Psychiatry, 22*(3), 463–471. https://doi.org/10.1002/wps.21122

Lusk, M., & Terrazas, S. (2015). Secondary trauma among caregivers who work with Mexican and Central American refugees. *Hispanic Journal of Behavioral Sciences, 37*(2), 257–273. https://doi.org/10.1177/0739986315578842

Lynch, S. H., & Lobo, M. L. (2012). Compassion fatigue in family caregivers: A Wilsonian concept analysis: Compassion fatigue. *Journal of Advanced Nursing, 68*(9), 2125–2134. https://doi.org/10.1111/j.1365-2648.2012.05985.x

Ma, L. M., & Penner, C. M. (2018). Tapestries of resilience: An arts-based approach to enhancing the resilience of World Vision's humanitarian staff. *Journal of Applied Arts & Health, 9*(2), 237–251. https://doi.org/10.1386/jaah.9.2.237_1

Mabingo, A. (2020). *Ubuntu as dance pedagogy in Uganda: Individuality, community, and inclusion in teaching and learning of indigenous dances.* Springer Nature.

Mackereth, P. A., White, K., Cawthorn, A., & Lynch, B. (2005). Improving stressful working lives: complementary therapies, counselling and clinical supervision for staff. *European Journal of Oncology Nursing, 9*(2), 147–154. https://doi.org/10.1016/j.ejon.2004.04.006

Magnuson, C. D., & Barnett, L. A. (2013). The playful advantage: How playfulness enhances coping with stress. *Leisure Sciences, 35*(2), 129–144. https://doi.org/10.1080/01490400.2013.761905

Main, M., & Solomon, J. (1990). Procedures for identifying infants as disorganized/disoriented during the Ainsworth Strange Situation. In M. T. Greenberg, D. Cicchetti, & E. M. Cummings (Eds.), *Attachment in the Preschool Years: Theory, Research, and Intervention* (pp. 121–160). University of Chicago Press.

Mangin, M., Sinha, R., & Fincher, K. (2014). Inflammation and vitamin D: The infection connection. *Inflammation Research, 63*(10), 803–819. https://doi.org/10.1007/s00011-014-0755-z

Mann, M., McMillan, J. E., Silver, E. J., & Stein, R. E. (2021). Children and adolescents with disabilities and exposure to disasters, terrorism, and the COVID-19 pandemic: A scoping review. *Current Psychiatry Reports, 23*(12), 1–12. https://doi.org/10.1007/s11920-021-01295-z

Marshall III, J. M. (2001). *The Lakota way: Stories and lessons for living. Native American wisdom on ethics and character.* Penguin Books.

Maslach, C., Jackson, S. E., & Leiter, M. (1996). *Maslach Burnout inventory manual* (3rd ed). Consulting Psychologists Press.

Mastandrea, S., Maricchiolo, F., Carrus, G., Giovannelli, I., Giuliani, V., & Berardi, D. (2018). Visits to figurative art museums may lower blood pressure and stress. *Arts Health, 5*, 1–10. doi: 10.1080/17533015.2018.1443953.

Masten, A. (2014). *Ordinary magic: Resilience in development.* Guilford Press.

Mateen, F. J. (2010). Neurological disorders in complex humanitarian emergencies and natural disasters. *Annals of Neurology, 68*(3), 282–294. https://doi.org/10.1002/ana.22135

McKay, L., & Barton, G. (2018). Exploring how arts-based reflection can support teachers' resilience and well-being. *Teaching and Teacher Education, 75*, 356–365. https://doi/org/10.1016/j.tate.2018.07.012

McMillan, J. M., & Jarvis, J. M. (2013). Mental health and students with disabilities: A review of literature. *Journal of Psychologists and Counsellors in Schools, 23*(2), 236–251. https://doi.org/10.1017/jgc.2013.14

Meehan, C. L., & Hawks, S. (2013). Cooperative breeding and attachment among the Aka foragers. In N. Quinn, & J. M. Mageo (Eds.), *Attachment reconsidered* (pp. 85–113). Palgrave Macmillan.

Menakem, R. (2017). *My grandmother's hands: Racialized trauma and the pathway to mending our hearts and bodies.* Penguin UK.

Merrill, S. M., Gladish, N., Fu, M. P., Moore, S. R., Konwar, C., Giesbrecht, G. F., MacIsaac, J. L., Kobor, M. S., & Letourneau, N. L. (2021). Associations of peripheral blood DNA methylation and estimated monocyte proportion differences during infancy with toddler attachment style. *Attachment & Human Development, 25*(1), 131–161. https://doi.org/10.1080/14616734.2021.1938872

Mesman, J., van Ijzendoorn, M., & Sagi-Schwartz, A. (2016). Cross cultural patterns of attachment. Universal and contextual dimensions. In J. Cassidy & P. Shaver (Eds.), *The handbook of attachment: theory, research, and clinical applications* (pp. 852–877). Guilford Press.

Michel, K. L. (2014, April 19). *Maslow's Hierarchy connected to Blackfoot beliefs.* A Digital Native American. Views of a Ho-Chunk journalist. https://lincolnmichel. wordpress.com/

Miranda, D. (2013). The role of music in adolescent development: Much more than the same old song. *International Journal of Adolescence and Youth, 18*(1), 5–22. https:// doi.org/1080/02673843.2011.650182

Mohr, E. (2014). Posttraumatic growth in youth survivors of a disaster: An arts-based research project. *Art Therapy, 31*(4), 155–162. https://doi.org/10.1080/07421 656.2015.963487

Monteiro, N. M., & Wall, D. J. (2011). African dance as healing modality throughout the diaspora: The use of ritual and movement to work through trauma. *The Journal of Pan African Studies, 4*(6), 234–252. https://link-gale-com.ezproxy2.library.drexel. edu/apps/doc/A306357808/AONE?u=drexel_main&sid=bookmark-AONE&xid= 3c56a9f2

Nagarajan, V. (2018). *Feeding a thousand souls: Women, ritual and ecology in India, An exploration of the Kōlam.* Oxford University Press.

Narayan, A. J., Rivera, L. M., Bernstein, R. E., Harris, W. W., & Lieberman, A. F. (2018). Positive childhood experiences predict less psychopathology and stress in pregnant women with childhood adversity: A pilot study of the benevolent childhood experiences (BCEs) scale. *Child Abuse & Neglect, 78*, 19–30. https://doi.org/10.1016/j.chi abu.2017.09.022

National Center for Complementary and Integrative Health. (2022). *Meditation and mindfulness: What you need to know.* National Institutes of Health. https://www.nccih. nih.gov/health/meditation-and-mindfulness-what-you-need-to-know

National Institute of Mental Health (2002). *Mental health and mass violence: Evidence-based early psychological intervention for victims/survivors of mass violence. A workshop to reach consensus on best practices.* NIH Publication No. 02-5138. U.S. Government Printing Office.

Neece, C. L., Green, S. A., & Baker, B. L. (2012). Parenting stress and child behavior problems: A transactional relationship across time. *American Journal on Intellectual and Developmental Disabilities, 117*(1), 48–66. https://doi.org/10.1352/ 1944-7558-117.1.48

Newman, B. M., & Newman, P. R. (2018). *Development through life: A psychosocial approach* (13th ed). Cengage Learning.

Ng, L. C., Kirk, C. M., Kanyanganzi, F., Fawzi, M. C. S., Sezibera, V., Shema, E., Bizimana, J. I., Cyamatare, F. R., & Betancourt, T. S. (2015). Risk and protective factors for suicidal ideation and behavior in Rwandan children. *British Journal of Psychiatry, 207*(3), 262–268. https://doi.org/10.1192/bjp.bp.114.154591

Nijs, L., & Nicolaou, G. (2021). Flourishing in resonance: Joint resilience building through music and motion. *Frontiers in Psychology*, *12*, 666702. https://doi.org/10.3389/fpsyg.2021.666702

Nobert, M., & Williamson, C. (2017). *Duty of care: Protection of humanitarian aid workers from sexual violence*. Report the Abuse. www.interaction.org/wp-content/uploads/resource-library/Report-the-Abuse_Duty-of-Care-Protection-of-Humanitarian-Aid-Workers-from-Sexual-Violence.pdf

Noble, K. G., Houston, S. M., Brito, N. H., Bartsch, H., Kan, E., Kuperman, J. M., Akshoomoff, N., Amaral, D. G., Bloss, C. S., Libiger, O., Schork, N. J., Murray, S. S., Casey, B. J., Chang, L., Ernst, T. M., Frazier, J. A., Gruen, J. R., Kennedy, D. N., Van Zijl, P. … Sowell, E. R. (2015). Family income, parental education and brain structure in children and adolescents. *Nature Neuroscience*, *18*(5), 773–778. https://doi.org/10.1038/nn.3983

Norman, R. E., Byambaa, M., De, R., Butchart, A., Scott, J., & Vos, T. (2012). The long-term health consequences of child physical abuse, emotional abuse, and neglect: A systematic review and meta-analysis. *PLoS Medicine*, *9*(11), 1–31. https://doi.org/10.1371/journal.pmed.1001349

Norris, F. H., Friedman, M. J., Watson, P. J., Byrne, C. M., Diaz, E., & Kaniasty, K. (2002). 60,000 disaster victims speak: Part I. An empirical review of the empirical literature, 1981–2001. *Psychiatry*, *65*(3), 207–239. https://doi.org/10.1521/psyc.65.3.207.20173

Nurullah, A. S. (2013). "It's really a roller coaster": Experience of parenting children with developmental disabilities. *Marriage & Family Review*, *49*(5), 412–445. https://doi.org/10.1080/01494929.2013.768320

Nutor, J. J., Duah, H. O., Agbadi, P., Duodu, P. A., & Gondwe, K. W. (2020). Spatial analysis of factors associated with HIV infection in Malawi: Indicators for effective prevention. *BMC Public Health*, *20*(1), 1167. https://doi.org/10.1186/s12889-020-09278-0

Opacin, N. (2020). *Peacebuilding education initiatives in a divided society: Dealing with the legacies of a violent past in Bosnia and Herzegovina* [Doctoral dissertation, RMIT University].

Operational Data Portal Refugee Statistics. (2023). *Uganda-refugee statistics Map-April 2023*. The UN Refugee Agency. https://data.unhcr.org/en/documents/details/100477

Orr, P. P. (2007). Art therapy with children after a disaster: A content analysis. *The Arts in Psychotherapy*, *34*(4), 350–361. https://doi.org/10.1016/j.aip.2007.07.002

Paardekooper, B., De Jong, J. T. V. M., & Hermanns, J. M. A. (1999). The psychological impact of war and the refugee situation on South Sudanese children in refugee camps in Northern Uganda: An exploratory study. *The Journal of Child Psychology and Psychiatry and Allied Disciplines*, *40*(4), 529–536. https://doi.org/10.1111/1469-7610.00471

Pacchiano, D., Connors, M., Klein, R., & Woodlock, K. (2021). Embedding workforce development into scaled innovations to prevent declines in administration quality. In J. A. List, D. Suskind & L. H. Supplee (Eds.), *The scale-up effect in early childhood and public policy: Why interventions lose impact at scale and what we can do about it* (pp. 350–369). Routledge.

Parten, M. B. (1932). Social participation among pre-school children. *The Journal of Abnormal and Social Psychology*, *27*(3), 243.

Pascoe, B. (2015). *The dark emu*. Magabala Books.

Pearlman, L. A., & Saakvitne, K.W. (1995). Treating therapists with vicarious traumatization and secondary traumatic stress disorders. In C. R. Figley (Ed.), *Compassion fatigue: Coping with secondary traumatic stress disorder in those who treat the traumatized*, (pp. 150–177). Brunner/Mazel.

Pederson, G. A., Smallegange, E., Coetzee, A., Hartog, K., Turner, J., Jordans, M. J. D., & Brown, F. L. (2019). A systematic review of the evidence for family and parenting interventions in low- and middle-income countries: Child and youth mental health outcomes. *Journal of Child and Family Studies, 28*, 2036–2055.

Pénzes, I., Engelbert, R., Heidendael, D., Oti, K., Jongen, E. M. M., & Hooren, S. V. (2023). The influence of art material and instruction during art making on brain activity: A quantitative electroencephalogram study. *The Arts in Psychotherapy, 83*, 102024. https://doi.org/10.1016/j.aip.2023.102024

Piaget, J. (2013). *Play, dreams and imitation in childhood*. Routledge.

Pielech, M., Sieberg, C. B., & Simons, L. E. (2013). Connecting parents of children with chronic pain through art therapy. *Clinical Practice in Pediatric Psychology, 1*(3), 214–226. https://doi.org/10.1037/cpp0000026

Pierson, R. (2013, May). *Every kid needs a champion* [Video]. TED Conferences. www.ted.com/talks/rita_pierson_every_kid_needs_a_champion

Pigni, A. (2016). *The idealist's survival kit: 75 simple ways to avoid burnout*. Parallax Press.

Pisani, L., Sabbagh, L., Salmoran, I., Mendoza, P., & Hommel, S. (2021). *HEART in Mexico city preschools: 2018–19 school year: Evaluation report*. Save the Children.

Pliske, M. M., Stauffer, S. D., & Werner-Lin, A. (2021). Healing from adverse childhood experiences through therapeutic powers of play: "I can do it with my hands". *International Journal of Play Therapy, 30*(4), 244–258. https://doi.org/10.1037/pla0000166

Poremski, D., Kuek, J. H. L., Yuan, Q., Li, Z., Yow, K. L., Eu, P. W., & Chua, H. C. (2022) The impact of peer support on the mental health of peer support specialists. *International Journal of Mental Health Systems, 16*(1), 1–51. https://doi.org/10.1186/s13033-022-00561-8

Potash, J. S., Yun Chen, J., & Yan Tsang, J. P. (2016). Medical student mandal making for holistic well-being. *Med Humanit., 42*(1), 17–25.

Poverty and Inequality Platform. (2022). *Country Profile*. The World Bank. https://pip.worldbank.org/country-profiles/MEX

Powell, S., Gómez-Carlier, N., & El-Halawani, M. (2021). Developing art therapy in the Arabian Gulf: Prioritizing relational models. In V. Huet & L. Kapitan (Eds.), *International advances in art therapy research and practice: The emerging picture* (pp. 168–176). Cambridge Scholars Publishing.

Proulx, L. (2002). Strengthening ties, parent-child-dyad: Group art therapy with toddlers and their parents. *American Journal of Art Therapy, 40*(4), 238–258.

Proyer, R. T. (2013). The well-being of playful adults: Adult playfulness, subjective well-being, physical well-being, and the pursuit of enjoyable activities. *European Journal of Humour Research, 1*(1), 84–98. https://doi.org/10.7592/EJHR2013.1.1.proyer

Proyer, R. T. (2014). Playfulness over the lifespan and its relation to happiness: Results from an online survey. *Zeitschrift für Gerontologie und Geriatrie, 47*(6), 508–512. https://doi.org/10.1007/s00391-013-0539-z

Proyer, R. T., Gander, F., Bertenshaw, E. J., & Brauer, K. (2018). The positive relationships of playfulness with indicators of health, activity, and physical fitness. *Frontiers
in Psychology*, *9*, 1440. https://doi.org/10.3389/fpsyg.2018.01440

Raskovic, Z., Obradovic, T. L., & Koprivica, I. (2019). *Supporting inclusion of children
with disabilities*: *Model of community-based services developed within the framework
of the Eastern European regional project "Community-based services for children
with disabilities."* Save the Children. https://resourcecentre.savethechildren.net/pdf/
Supporting-Inclusion-of-Children-with-Disabilities.-Model-of-Community-Based-
Services.pdf/

Rasmitadila, R., Aliyyah, R. R., Rachmadtullah, R., Samsudin, A., Syaodih, E., Nurtanto,
M., & Tambunan, A. R. S. (2020). The perceptions of primary school teachers of online
learning during the COVID-19 pandemic period. *Journal of Ethnic and Cultural
Studies*, *7*(2), 90–109. https://doi.org/10.29333/ejecs/388

Reed, R. V., Fazel, M., Jones, L., Panter-Brick, C., & Stein, A. (2012). Mental health
of displaced and refugee children resettled in low-income and middle-income countries: Risk and protective factors. *The Lancet*, *379*(9812), 250–265. https://doi.org/
10.1016/S0140-6736(11)60050-0

Regehr, C., & Cadell, S. (1999). Secondary trauma in sexual assault crisis
work: Implications for therapists and therapy. *Canadian Social Work*, *1*, 56–70.

Reilly, R. (2010). Disabilities among refugees and conflict-affected populations. *Forced
Migration Review*, (35), 8–10.

Reser, D., Simmons, M., Johns, E., Ghaly, A., Quayle, M., Dordevic, A. L., Tare, M.,
McArdle, A., Willems, J., Yunkaporta, T & Suppiah, V. (2021). Australian Aboriginal
techniques for memorization: Translation into a medical and allied health education
setting. *PloS One*, *16*(5), e0251710. https://doi.org/10.1371/journal.pone.0251710

Roome, E., Raven, J., & Martineau, T. (2014). Human resource management in post-
conflict health systems: Review of research and knowledge gaps. *Conflict and Health*,
8(1), 1–12. https://doi.org/10.1186/1752-1505-8-18

Rose, D. H., & Meyer, A. (2002). *Teaching every student in the digital age: Universal
design for learning*. Association for Supervision and Curriculum Development.

Rubin, J. A. (2005). *Child art therapy* (25th ed.). John Wiley & Sons, Inc.

Rubin, J. A. (2010). *Introduction to art therapy: Sources & resources* (2nd ed.).
Routledge. https://doi.org/10.4324/9780203893968

Rubin, J. A. (2012). *Approaches to art therapy: Theory and technique*. Routledge.

Runco, M. A. (2014). *Creativity: Theories and themes: Research, development, and
practice* (2nd ed.). Elsevier Academic Press.

Runco, M. A., & Jaeger, G. J. (2012). The standard definition of creativity. *Creativity
Research Journal*, *24*(1), 92–96. https://doi.org/10.1080/10400419.2012.650092

Ruppert, S. S. (2006). How the arts benefit student achievement. Retrieved on August 16,
2023 from https://eric.ed.gov/?id=ED529766.

Russ, S. W. (2016). Pretend play: Antecedent of adult creativity. *New Directions for
Child and Adolescent Development*, *151*, 21–32. https://doi.org/10.1002/cad.20154

Russ, S. W., & Wallance, C. E. (2013). Pretend play and the creative process. *American
Journal of Play*, *6*(1), 136–148.

Samplin, E., Ikuta, T., Malhotra, A. K., Szeszko, P. R., & DeRosse, P. (2013). Sex
differences in resilience to childhood maltreatment: Effects of trauma history on

hippocampal volume, general cognition, and subclinical psychosis in healthy adults. *Journal of Psychiatric Research, 47*(9),1174–1179. https://doi.org/10.1016/j.jpsychi res.2013.05.008

Sarkissian, A. D., & Sharkey, J. D. (2021). Transgenerational trauma and mental health needs among Armenian genocide descendants. *Int. J. Environ. Res. Public Health, 18*(9), 10554.

Save the Children. (2017). *Baseline study of attitudes and knowledge of the children with disability issue.*

Save the Children. (2019a). *Final evaluation of community-based services for children with disabilities project.*

Save the Children. (2019b). *HEART in Bosnia and Herzegovina – 2019 Annual Program Report.*

Save the Children. (2020). *When am I going to start to live?: The urgent need to repatriate foreign children trapped in Al Hol and Roj Camps* www.savethechildren.org/cont ent/dam/usa/reports/emergency-response/when-am-i-going-to-start-to-live-report.pdf

Save the Children. (2021a). *Evaluation report – Impact of HEART Program implementation on children in Georgia's early and preschool education settings.* Save the Children International Georgia.

Save the Children. (2021b). *HEART safe back to school Malawi report: The use of HEART in the transition back to primary school after COVID-19 lockdown.*

Save the Children. (2021c). *HEART in Uganda – 2021 program report.*

Save the Children. (2021d). *When am I going to start to live?: The urgent need to repatriate foreign children trapped in Al Hol and Roj Camps.*

Save the Children. (2022a). *HEART in Uganda – 2022 program report.*

Save the Children. (2022b). *Internal monitoring report – Mental health and psychosocial support program.* Save the Children Indonesia.

Save the Children. (2023a). *Global survey report: Reflections on personal experience in HEART training participation.*

Save the Children. (2023b). *Interview report: Experiences of the Healing and Education Through the Arts (HEART).* Donor Champion Charlene Engelhard.

Save the Children. (2023c). *Parent caregiver peer support group MEAL report: Results of a program pilot in Lebanon and Syria.* Internal Program Monitoring Report.

Save the Children. (2023d). *Participant reflections on staff peer support groups in the United States.* Internal Report.

Schalock, R. L., Luckasson, R., & Tassé, M. J. (2019). The contemporary view of intellectual and developmental disabilities: Implications for psychologists. *Psicothema, 31*(3), 223–228. https://doi.org/10.7334/psicothema2019.119

Schininà, G., Hosn, M. A., Ataya, A., Dieuveut, K., & Salem, M. A. (2010). Psychosocial response to the Haiti earthquake: The experiences of International Organization for Migration. *Intervention Journal of Mental Health and Psychosocial Support in Conflict Affected Areas, 8*(2), 158–164. https://doi.org/10.1097/WTF.0b013e32833c2f78

Selye, H. (1951). *The physiology and pathology of exposure to stress: A treatise based on the concepts of the general-adaptation-syndrome and the diseases of adaptation.* Montreal, Acta.

Seymour, H. A. (n.d.). *The philosophy of music: What music can do for you.* Pranava Books. (Original work published 1920).

Seymour, S. C. (2013). "It takes a village to raise a child": Attachment theory and multiple childcare in Alor, Indonesia, and in North India. In N. Quinn, & J.M. Mageo (Eds.), *Attachment reconsidered* (pp. 115–139). Palgrave Macmillan.

Shaturaev, J. (2021). A comparative analysis of public education system of Indonesia and Uzbekistan. *Bioscience Biotechnology Research Communications*, *14*(5), 89–92. https://doi.org/10.21786/bbrc/14.5/18

Shen, X. (2023). Play and scientific creativity: A critical review and an integrative theoretical framework. *The Journal of Creative Behavior*, *57*(4), 503–515. https://doi.org/10.1002/jocb.596

Shen, X., Chick, G., & Pitas, N. A. (2017). From playful parents to adaptable children: A structural equation model of the relationships between playfulness and adaptability among young adults and their parents. *International Journal of Play*, *6*(3), 244–254. https://doi.org/10.1080/21594937.2017.1382983

Shonkoff, J. P. (2010). Building a new biodevelopmental framework to guide the future of early childhood policy. *Child Development*, *81*(1), 357–367. https://doi.org/10.1111/j.1467-8624.2009.01399.x

Shonkoff, J. P., & Garner, A. S. (2011). The lifelong effects of early childhood adversity and toxic stress. *Pediatrics*, *129*(1), e232–246. https://doi.org/10.1542/peds.2011-2663

Shore, A. (2013). *The practitioner's guide to child art therapy: Fostering creativity and relational growth*. Routledge.

Siddique, C. M., & D'Arcy, C. (1984). Adolescence, stress, and psychological well-being. *Journal of Youth and Adolescence*, *13*(6), 459–473. https://doi.org/10.1007/BF02088593

Silver, R. (2000) *Developing cognitive and creative skills through art*. Ablin Press.

Singer, D. G., Singer, J. L., Plaskon, S. L., & Schweder, A. E. (2003). A role for play in the preschool curriculum. In S. Olfman (Ed.), *All work and no play ... How educational reforms are harming our preschoolers* (pp. 43–70). Praeger Publishers/Greenwood Publishing Group.

Singha, S., Warr, M., Mishra, P. & Henriksen, D. (2020). Playing with creativity across the lifespan: A conversation with Dr. Sandra Russ. *TechTrends*, *64*, 550–554. https://doi.org/10.1007/s11528-020-00514-3

Skeen, S., Macedo, A., Tomlinson, M., Hensels, I. S., & Sherr, L. (2016). Exposure to violence and psychological well-being over time in children affected by HIV/AIDS in South Africa and Malawi. *AIDS Care*, *28*(sup1), 16–25. https://doi.org/10.1080/09540121.2016.1146219

Slopen, N., Shonkoff, J. P., Albert, M. A., Yoshikawa, H., Jacobs, A., Stoltz, R., & Williams, D. R. (2016). Racial disparities in child adversity in the US: Interactions with family immigration history and income. *American Journal of Preventive Medicine*, *50*(1), 47–56. https://doi.org/10.1016/j.amepre.2015.06.013

Smilansky, S. (1968). *The effects of sociodramatic play on disadvantaged preschool children*. Wiley.

Smith, P. K. (1978). A longitudinal study of social participation in preschool children: Solitary and parallel play reexamined. *Developmental Psychology*, *14*(5), 517–523. https://doi.org/10.1037/0012-1649.14.5.517

Snyder, K., Malhotra, B., & Kaimal, G. (2021). Team value and visual voice: Healthcare providers perspectives on the contributions and impact of art therapy in pediatric hematology/oncology clinics. *The Arts in Psychotherapy, 75*, 101808. https://doi.org/10.1016/j.aip.2021.101808

Solis, S. L., Liu, C. W., & Popp, J. M. (2020). *Learning to cope through play: Playful learning as an approach to support children's coping during times of heightened stress and adversity.* The LEGO Foundation. https://cms.learningthroughplay.com/media/jqifsynb/learning-to-cope-through-play.pdf

Spirito, A., Stark, L. J., Grace, N., & Stamoulis, D. (1991). Common problems and coping strategies reported in childhood and early adolescence. *Journal of Youth and Adolescence, 20*(5), 531–544. https://doi.org/10.1007/BF01540636

Stough, L. M., Ducy, E. M., & Kang, D. (2017). Addressing the needs of children with disabilities experiencing disaster or terrorism. *Current Psychiatry Reports, 19*(4), 24. https://doi.org/10.1007/s11920-017-0776-8

Suffren, S., La Buissonnière-Ariza, V., Tucholka, A., Nassim, M., Séguin, J. R., Boivin, M., Kaur Singh, M., Foland-Ross, L. C., Leope, F., Gotlib, I. H., Tremblay, R. E. & Maheu, F. S. (2021). Prefrontal cortex and amygdala anatomy in youth with persistent levels of harsh parenting practices and subclinical anxiety symptoms over time during childhood. *Development and Psychopathology, 34*(3), 1–12. https://doi.org/10.1017/S0954579420001716

Taleb, N. N. (2014). *Antifragile: Things that gain from disorder* (Incerto). Random House Incorporated.

Taylor, A. F., & Butts-Wilmsmeyer, C. (2020). Self-regulation gains in kindergarten relatedto frequency of green schoolyard use. *Journal of Environmental Psychology, 70*, 101440. https://doi.org/10.1016/j.jenvp.2020.101440

Tedeschi, R. G., & Calhoun, L. G. (1996). The post traumatic growth inventory: Measuring the positive legacy of trauma. *Journal of Traumatic Stress, 9*(3), 455–471. https://doi.org/10.1002/jts.2490090305

Teicher, M. H., & Parigger, A. (2015). The "Maltreatment and Abuse Chronology of Exposure" (MACE) scale for the retrospective assessment of abuse and neglect during development. *PLoS One, 10*(2), e0117423. https://doi.org/10.1371/journal.pone.0117423

Terranova, A. M., Boxer, P., & Morris, A. S. (2009). Factors influencing the course of posttraumatic stress following a natural disaster: Children's reactions to Hurricane Katrina. *Journal of Applied Developmental Psychology, 30*(3), 344–355. https://doi.org/10.1016/j.appdev.2008.12.017

Thergaonkar, N., & Daniel, D. (2019). Effect of arts based therapy on functionality of children with intellectual disability. *Journal of Indian Association for Child and Adolescent Mental Health, 15*(2), 55–71. https://doi.org/10.1177/0973134220190204

Thompson, G. (2012). Family-centered music therapy in the home environment: Promoting interpersonal engagement between children with autism spectrum disorder and their parents. *Music Therapy Perspectives, 30*(2), 109–116. https://doi.org/10.1093/mtp/30.2.109

Tierney, A. L., & Nelson, C. A. (2009) Brain development and the role of experience in the early years. *Zero to Three, 30*(2), 9–13.

Tol, W. A., Komproe, I. H., Susanty, D., Jordans, M. J., Macy, R. D., & De Jong, J. T. (2008). School-based mental health intervention for children affected by political violence in Indonesia: a cluster randomized trial. *JAMA, 300*(6), 655–662. https://doi.org/10.1001/jama.300.6.655

Tomoda, A., Polcari, A., Anderson, C. M., Teicher, M. H., & Huang, H. (2012). Reduced visual cortex gray matter volume and thickness in young adults who witnessed domesticviolence during childhood. *PLoS One, 7*(12), e52528. https://doi.org/10.1371/journal.pone.0052528

Touloumakos, A. K., & Barrable, A. (2020) Adverse childhood experiences: The protective and therapeutic potential of nature. *Frontiers in Psychology, 11*, 597935. https://doi.org/10.3389/fpsyg.2020.597935

Udwin, O., Boyle, S., Yule, W., Bolton, D., & O'Ryan, D. (2000). Risk factors for longterm psychological effects of a disaster experienced in adolescence: Predictors of post traumatic stress disorder. *The Journal of Child Psychology and Psychiatry and Allied Disciplines, 41*(8), 969–979. https://doi.org/10.1111/1469-7610.00685

Ugurlu, N., Akca, L., & Acarturk, C. (2016). An art therapy intervention for symptoms of post-traumatic stress, depression and anxiety among Syrian refugee children. *Vulnerable Children and Youth Studies, 11*(2), 89–102. https://doi.org/10.1080/17450128.2016.1181288

United Nations. (2006). Convention on the Rights of Persons with Disabilities.

United Nations Children's Fund. (2005). *Violence against disabled children: UN Secretary Generals report on violence against children thematic group on violence against disabled children: Findings and recommendations.* https://discovery.ucl.ac.uk/id/eprint/15686/1/15686.pdf

United Nations Children's Fund. (2016). *Children in humanitarian crises: What business can do.* https://unglobalcompact.org/library/4671

United Nations Children's Fund. (2017a, December 25). *All children in Georgia should have equal access to quality early and pre-school education, UNICEF says* [Press release]. www.unicef.org/georgia/press-releases/all-children-georgia-should-have-equal-access-quality-early-and-pre-school-education

United Nations Children's Fund. (2017b, December 7). *Social services for children with disabilities in Georgia are scarce and a lot of children are barred from realizing their rights, UNICEF says* [Press release]. www.unicef.org/georgia/press-releases/social-services-children-disabilities-georgia-are-scarce-and-lot-children-are-barred

United Nations Children's Fund. (2017). *Protecting the Rights of the Child in Humanitarian Situations: Report of the United Nations High Commissioner for human rights.* https://digitallibrary.un.org/record/3843475?ln=en

United Nations Children's Fund. (2019). *A world ready to learn: Prioritizing quality each childhood education. Global Report.* https://www.unicef.org/media/57926/file/A-world-ready-to-learn-advocacy-brief-2019.pdf

United Nations Children's Fund. (2021). *Seen, counted, included: Using data to shed light on the well-being of children with disabilities.* https://data.unicef.org/resources/children-with-disabilities-report-2021/

United Nations Department of Economic and Social Affairs. (2016, February 8). *Disability-inclusive humanitarian action.* https://www.un.org/development/desa/disabilities/news/news/disability-inclusive-humanitarian action.html

United Nations Humanitarian Needs Assessment Program Syria. (2021). *Disability in Syria: Investigation on the intersectional impacts of gender, age and a decade of conflict on persons with disabilities.* https://www.hi-deutschland-projekte.de/lnob/wp-content/uploads/sites/2/2021/09/hnap-disability-in-syria-investigation-on-intersectional-impacts-2021.pdf

United Nations Office for the Coordination of Humanitarian Affairs. (2019, March). *OCHA duty of care framework: Version 12.* https://resourcecenter.undac.org/wp-content/uploads/2021/01/OCHA-Duty-of-Care-Framework_PSMC-endorsed.pdf

United Nations Office on Drugs and Crime. (2018). *Angola.* https://dataunodc.un.org/content/country-list

United Nations Office on Drugs and Crime. (2019).*Global study on homicide.* https://www.unodc.org/unodc/en/data-and-analysis/global-study-on-homicide.html

United Nations Office of Drugs and Crime (2023). *Global study on homicide: 2023.* https://www.unodc.org/documents/data-and-analysis/gsh/2023/Global_study_on_homicide_2023_web.pdf

United Nations Population Fund (2022). *World population dashboard Indonesia.* https://www.unfpa.org/data/world-population/ID.

UNHCR, The UN Refugee Agency. (2023a). Global trends: Forced displacement in 2022. www.unhcr.org/global-trends-report-2022

UNHCR, The UN Refugee Agency. (2023). Refugees and asylum Seekers in Uganda: Uganda refugee response. https://data.unhcr.org/en/documents/details/100477

U.S. Department of Health and Human Services. (n.d.). *HIV and AIDS and mental health.* National Institute of Mental Health. https://www.nimh.nih.gov/health/topics/hiv-aids

Vallières, F., Hyland, P., McAuliffe, E., Mahmud, I., Tulloch, O., Walker, P., & Taegtmeyer, M. (2018). A new tool to measure approaches to supervision from the perspective of community health workers: a prospective, longitudinal, validation study in seven countries. *BMC Health Services Research, 18*(1), 1–8. https://doi.org/10.1186/s12913-018-3595-7

van Dernoot Lipsky, L., & Burk, C. (2009). *Trauma stewardship: An everyday guide to caring for self while caring for others.* Berrett-Koehler Publishers.

Vaughan, T., & Caldwell, B. J. (2017). Impact of the creative arts indigenous parental engagement (CAIPE) program. *Australian Art Education, 38*(1), 76–92.

Vik, S., & Somby, H. M. (2018). Defectology and inclusion. *Issues in Early Education, 42*(3), 94–102. https://doi.org/10.26881/pwe.2018.42.10

von der Assen, N., Euwema, M., & Cornielje, H. (2010). Including disabled children in psychosocial programmes in areas affected by armed conflict. *Intervention, 8*(1), 29–39. https://doi.org/10.1097/WTF.0b013e328338561a

Vygotsky, L. (1978). *Mind in society.* Harvard University Press.

Wadende, P., Morara, A., & Oburu, P.O. (2016). African indigenous care-giving practices: Stimulating early childhood development and education in Kenya. *South African Journal of Childhood Education, 6*(2), 1–7. https://doi.org/10.4102/sajce.v6i2.446

Westwood, P. (2011). *Commonsense methods for students with special educational needs* (6th ed.) Routledge.

Wico, D. M., Huber, T., & Schnyder, S. S. (2021). Theater arts as a beneficial and educational venue in identifying and providing therapeutic coping skills for early childhood adversities: A systematic review of the literature. *International Electronic Journal of Elementary Education, 13*(4), 457–467. https://doi.org/10.26822/iejee.2021.204

Wordsworth, D. (2017, April 27). *The refugee rethink part 4: What if Maslow was wrong?*. Medium: Becoming Alight. https://medium.com/becoming-alight/the-refugee-rethink-part-4-what-if-maslow-was-wrong-27eb49707548

The World Bank (2016). *The World Bank in Syrian Arab Republic.* www.worldbank.org/en/country/syria/overview

The World Bank. (2022a). *Country profile: Mexico.* https://pip.worldbank.org/country-profiles/MEX

The World Bank. (2022b). *The World Bank in Lebanon.* www.worldbank.org/en/country/lebanon/overview

The World Bank (2022c). *The World Bank in Syrian Arab Republic.* www.worldbank.org/en/country/syria/overview

The World Bank (2023a). *Poverty and Equity Brief: Mexico.* https://pip.worldbank.org/country-profiles/MEX

The World Bank (2023b). *Poverty and Equity Brief: Georgia.* https://pip.worldbank.org/country-profiles/GEO

World Health Organization. (2008). *Maternal mental health and child health and development in low and middle income countries: Report of the meeting, Geneva, Switzerland, 30 January–1 February, 2008.* www.who.int/publications/i/item/9789241597142

World Health Organization. (2020). *Mental health.* www.who.int/news-room/fact-sheets/detail/mental-health-strengthening-our-response

World Health Organization. (2022). *World mental health report: Transforming mental health for all.* https://iris.who.int/bitstream/handle/10665/356119/9789240049338-eng.pdf?isAllowed=y&sequence=1

World Health Organization & World Bank. (2011). *World report on disability 2011.* World Health Organization. https://apps.who.int/iris/handle/10665/44575

Yarrow, N., Masood, E., & Afkar, R. (2020). *Estimated impacts of COVID-19 on learning and earning in Indonesia: How to turn the tide.* International Bank for Reconstruction and Development/The World Bank. https://openknowledge.worldbank.org/server/api/core/bitstreams/fe106b4f-edf3-5f1b-9272-7c52136edef0/content

Yogman, M., Garner, A., Hutchinson, J., Hirsh-Pasek, K., & Golinkoff, R. M. (2018). The power of play: A pediatric role in enhancing development in young children. *Pediatrics, 142*(3), e20182058. https://doi.org/10.1542/peds.2018-2058

Zeanah, C. H., Humphreys, K. L., Fox, N. A., & Nelson, C. A. (2017). Alternatives for abandoned children: Insights from the Bucharest Early Intervention Project. *Current Opinion in Psychology, 15,* 182–188. https://doi.org/10.1016/j.copsyc.2017.02.024

Glossary

Antifragility: The capacity to become strengthened rather than defeated by adversity.

Adverse Childhood Experience (ACE) An extremely stressful or potentially traumatic event that occurs in childhood and youth.

Attachment The emotional relationship between the child and caregiver or between two individuals in a relationship.

Anxious Attachment Response to intrusive or alternately caring and harsh parenting that keeps a child, and eventual adult, worried about the status and safety of the relationship.

Avoidant Attachment A response to neglect and abandonment in the parent child relationship that results in an individual being avoidant of intimacy and interdependence.

Bilateral Donor A governmental agency that provides funding from one country to another, often to support global development or humanitarian response.

Burnout A condition that develops gradually and can lead to emotional exhaustion, depersonalization, and reduced personal accomplishment that can occur among individuals who work with people in conditions of chronic stress or distress.

Compassion Fatigue A state of overall dysfunction and exhaustion of biological, psychological, and social well-being that develops as a result of caring for people in significant emotional and/or physical distress.

Compassion Satisfaction The pleasure derived from effectively helping others as well as a sense of efficacy in one's ability to make a positive impact on the world. It is considered a protective factor against compassion fatigue.

COVID-19 A respiratory illness caused by the SARS-CoV-2 virus which was declared as a pandemic by the World Health Organization in 2020, which led to widespread health, social, and economic impacts across the globe.

Chronosystem The part of the ecological systems theory that focuses on changes over time and the ever-changing dynamic environment involving life changes and social issues.

Cultural Semiotic Systems The symbolic representation of knowledge through drawing pictures, reading, writing, maps, and diagrams.

Disaster A significant adverse event caused by natural phenomena (such as earthquakes, tsunamis, hurricanes) or human activities (such as armed conflicts).

Disorganized Attachment The interpersonal response to abusive early childhood contexts where the child is unable to form any stable sense of relationships with caregivers or peers (another term for fearful attachment).

Distress Pain or suffering affecting the body or the mind.

Ecological Systems Theory The idea that we as human beings are part of a system of expanding networks of relationships that affect the course of our life trajectories.

Emotion-Focused Strategies Include strategies that help to reduce negative emotional responses associated with stress, especially when the sources of stress are not changeable. Examples can include cognitive reframing, distraction and relaxation, meditation, or art making.

Eustress A positive form of stress having a beneficial effect on health, motivation, performance, and/or emotional well-being.

Exosystem The part of the ecological systems theory that includes settings that may not contain children but affect them, such as their parents' workplaces, religious institutions, and community health services.

Fearful Attachment Response to profoundly abusive early childhood contexts where the child is unable to form any stable sense of relationships with caregivers or peers (another term for disorganized attachment).

GABA Abbreviation for Gamma aminobutyric acid, a time of neurotransmitter.

Global Development A broad term used for the field of promoting human and economic development, including the reduction of poverty, for countries and regions around the world.

HEART Acronym for the Save the Children's Healing and Education through the Arts program.

Humanitarian Response The field of global work that responds to the human and economic needs resulting from an emergency such as a natural disaster or armed conflict.

Humanitarian Workers Professional workers who assist people in conditions of adversity. They can be from local populations including the affected community, or international (from outside the affected community).

Inclusive Education Educational approaches that enable all children to learn together, with support for their individual needs.

INGO Acronym for International Non-Governmental Organization.

Macrosystem The part of the ecological systems theory that impacts individuals and communities based on the values, laws, customs, and culture that surround them.

Mental Health   A state of well-being in which an individual can realize their own abilities, cope with stress, and productively engage in their community.

MHPSS   Acronym for Mental Health and Psychosocial Support.

Mesosystem   The part of the ecological systems theory focused on the connections between a child's microsystems, such as interactions between family members from home and teachers or friends at school.

Mindfulness   Awareness of being in the present moment including efforts to reflect on one's thoughts and feelings without judgment.

Microsystem   The part of the ecological systems theory which includes the impact of and dynamics within the relations between a child and others in their immediate environment such as friends, family members, teachers, and other caregivers.

Multilateral Donor   An international organization that pools funding from multiple countries (including governments) to collectively support global development or humanitarian response.

Neuroplasticity   The idea that the brain functions via neural connections and pathways and that these pathways can be consistently modified and updated by new experiences.

Nexus Setting   Refers to a location in which there is ongoing or recurrent transition between humanitarian and development programming.

Operational Stressors   Types of stressors inherent in humanitarian work, such as working long hours, exposure to adversities, and working and living in a stressful environment.

Organizational Stressors   Stressors related to a particular humanitarian organization such as workplace culture and organizational structure.

PACEs: Acronym for Protective And Compensatory Experiences.

Parent/Caregiver (PCG)   Any person with whom the child normally lives and who provides daily care to the child such as biological parents, adoptive parents with parental rights, or biological family members such as grandparents or older siblings.

People with Disabilities   Individuals with physical, intellectual, mental, or sensory impairments which may hinder their full and effective participation in society.

Primary Schools   Educational institutions providing the first stage of compulsory education, typically for students aged 5–12 years.

Preschools   Educational institutions providing pre-primary education that supports the early learning and development of children often aged 3–5 years.

Post-Traumatic Growth (PTG)   Refers to positive psychological changes that some people have after experiencing a traumatic event that leads to a new way of life by building on existing and newly identified strengths. PTG is associated with adaptive transformations occur after a traumatic experience by building on existing and newly identified strengths.

PTSD   Acronym for post-traumatic stress disorder

Problem-Focused Strategies   Refers to strategies to address stressful situations in an active and direct manner.

Protective and Compensatory Experiences (PACEs)   Refers to experiences that offset the negative impacts of adversities and make them manageable or help reduce the damage they might cause. These can include fulfilling activities and supportive relationships and entities.

Psychosocial Support   Actions and approaches that address the psychological and social needs of individuals, families, and communities.

Resilience   The ability to return to how things were or the ability to bounce back from challenges.

Secondary Traumatic Stress (STS)   A stress reaction resulting from knowledge about a traumatic event experienced by another person.

Self-Care   The ability to care for oneself in ways that promote physical and mental well-being.

Sign Systems   Symbolic representation of knowledge through drawing, reading, writing, maps, and diagrams.

Sociocultural Theory   Theory that explores the way that culture is transmitted from one generation to the next.

Secondary Schools   Educational Institutions that provide post-primary education, typically for students aged 12–18 years of age.

Stress   The mental and physical response resulting from exposure to pressure or adverse conditions.

Third Country National   A person in a process of migration who is in transit, currently not their country of origin, waiting to travel to another country that is also not their country of origin.

Toxic Positivity   A dysfunctional response to recognizing and managing emotions by promoting positive emotions while ignoring negative ones.

Traumatic Event   An extremely distressing event that is outside of normal human experience.

Vicarious Trauma   Stress, distress, or traumatic response that results from exposure to the traumatic experiences of others.

Vicarious Resilience   The positive aspects of working to support people affected by adversity, including those that have experienced stressful, distressful, or traumatic events, often deriving from exposure to their personal strength, growth, and recovery.

Zone of Proximal Development   The difference between what children can do alone and what they can do through collaboration with, and guidance from, peers and/or adults.

Appendix

This section offers an overview on theories of maturation from childhood to youth in terms of physiological, socio-emotional, cognitive, and artistic development.

Physiological, Socio-emotional, and Cognitive Development

A child's physical development from birth through childhood and youth is impacted by many factors including genetics and the environment. The developmental milestones typically involve a process of gross motor to fine motor aspects. This unfolding of physical milestones involves a series of physical attributes like rolling over, crawling, walking, and running. Children go from learning to regulate and manage their whole bodies to gaining increasing control over their extremities and digits although this process can be delayed or disrupted for children with some types of chronic health conditions and/or disabilities. These physical developments are influenced by nurturance in the environment, including the physical qualities of the air, water, food, and nutrition, as well as the responses to threats and stress through emotional support. As children mature and grow in their bodies, a major milestone is the approach of puberty which results in the development of primary and secondary sexual characteristics. These changes result in hormonal changes for girls and boys leading to brain and body maturation to adulthood. Girls tend to grow for a few more years after menarche while boys tend to grow physically late into their teenage years. Both boys' and girls' brains develop fully only by about age 25 which is when their ability for judgment and decision making are most like an adult.

Along with social and emotional development, this increasing pattern of differentiation and complexity in thinking occurs as part of cognitive development. Based on close observations of children including his own, theorist Jean Piaget proposed a stage model of cognitive development between infancy and adulthood. He recognized that children experience changes in distinct stages and actively develop knowledge as they explore their world (Berk, 2019). These stages include sensorimotor (0–2 years), pre-operational (2–7 years), concrete operational (7–11 years), and formal operational (11 years to adulthood). According to him, two processes are key to cognitive development – *accommodation* – the process of adapting cognitive schemes of viewing the world that fit reality; and *assimilation* – interpreting experiences in terms of familiar cognitive schemes (Goswami, 2008). Piaget has been criticized for overemphasizing the cultural universality of his stage theory, underestimating the role of experience and culture. Moreover, research has shown that development is more continuous and that there is considerable overlap among the four stages rather than the stages being qualitatively different and hierarchical (Crain, 2015).

Once the child is aware of self and able to complete basic functions like eating, drinking, basic language, and self-care, they are increasingly aware of and able to distinguish between themselves and others. They move from being ego centric (focused on themselves and their own needs) to becoming aware of others including that other humans and living beings have their own thoughts, feelings, and perspectives and is an essential milestone for children to be both individuals as well as interconnected members of their families and communities. The way this develops in the form of attachments to others, sets the stage for life.

The theories summarized above are commonly taught to healthcare and education professionals. Less widely known are the developmental theories around creative and artistic development and the stages of play. The next section provides an overview of stages of development in visual arts, music, and dance and movement as well as play.

Stages of Development in the Realms of Visual Arts, Music, Dance and Movement

Visual Artistic Development

Seminal work by Lowenfeld and Brittain (1987) outlined distinct stages of drawing development in children. In the Scribble Stage (ages 2–4), the child's marks progress from disordered lines to more controlled movements, and eventually named scribbles, indicating growth in motor skills. Next is the Preschematic Stage (ages 4–7) in which a "head-feet representation of a person" typically develops and the child typically draws "objects in their environment with which they have had contact," indicating growth in conceptual organization and awareness (Lowenfeld & Brittain, 1987). During this stage, drawings can appear random in size and orientation on the page and children are typically excited to discuss their representations with others. During the Schematic Stage (ages 7–9), the child displays assimilation of external factors and intellectual growth as objects appear "in a straight line across the bottom of the page" (known as a baseline). The child also develops a schema for various objects and repeatedly draws each object in the same way. In the Stage of Dawning Realism (9–12 years), drawings are more focused on symbolism than on representation, and children are often more self-conscious about their artwork. Finally, the Pseudo-Naturalistic Stage (beginning at approximately age 11 or 12) reflects growth in individualization and social relationships. During this stage, children often exhibit more self-consciousness with artwork and greater awareness of sexual characteristics in drawings.

How similar or different are these stages in Visual Artistic Development? According to Lowenfeld and Brittain (1987), the "natural development of a youngster does not extend beyond this stage," but if the child chooses to continue artistic education, they can acquire greater skills. Lowenfeld claimed that these stages of artistic development occurred regardless of where the child was geographically located, though this notion is beginning to be investigated and challenged (Goodman et al., 2022). Questions about whether children experience the same artistic developmental stages across the globe have begun to be explored. In their research of drawings from a play-based intervention in Ugandan preschools, Goodman et al. (2022) found that as opposed to the horizontal baseline noted by Lowenfeld and Brittain (1987), most of the artwork by Ugandan preschoolers in their sample exhibited vertical baselines. Therefore, they wrote: "Lowenfeld's rarely challenged baseline theory must be revisited critically" (Goodman et al., 2022). When looking at similarities and differences between children's artistic development across various cultural groups, there needs to be further study to "address global influences that are manifest through a broad spectrum of socioculturally learned behaviors, deeply rooted expectations, and robust media trends" (Goodman et al., 2022).

American art therapist Judith Rubin sought to create a stage-approach to artistic development that did not only focus on drawing but also painting and creating sculptural forms (Rubin, 2005). As the child grows fine and gross motor control as well as access to different materials, they exhibit more control over how they manipulate these materials including representing, symbols, personal style, and critical reflection of their own work. Art therapist Rawley Silver (2000) explored variations in children's artwork when working with children who experienced physical and cognitive disabilities. She outlined four objectives in approaching art in an open-ended way: widening the range of communication, inviting exploratory learning, providing tasks that are self-rewarding, and reinforcing emotional balance (Silver, 2000). Through her research, she made observations that "drawings can serve as instruments for identifying and evaluating cognitive skills that are usually associated with language" and that "art procedures that emphasize communication, adjustment, enjoyment, and exploratory learning can help children with communication disorders and children with learning disabilities develop concepts of space, order, and class" (p. 236). Another scholar, Rhoda Kellogg, collected over a million drawings by children from around the world and developed her theory of artistic development in children. She noted that globally, children begin scribbling around age 2, on paper with a crayon, in the dirt with a stick, and in the sand with a shell.

She stated that these scribbles are the building blocks of children's art (Kellogg & O'Dell, 1967).

Musical Development

Over a century ago, Harriet Ayer Seymour's (n.d./1920) groundbreaking work discussed the benefits of providing children with a musical environment in the home. Since then, multiple theories on musical development in children have been created, and a number are mentioned below. Notably, variations in the types of tasks required for typical musical developmental milestones (skill learning, rhythm learning, tonal learning, and pattern learning) can require differences in developmental timelines (Gordon, 2012). Bruscia (1991) identified the following model of typical musical developmental stages, beginning before birth: the amniotic period, descending the birth canal, birth, 0–6 months, 6–24 months, 2–7 years, 7–12 years, 12–18 years, and 18 years and above. He identified the amniotic period as being the primary musical experience as the fetus is exposed to sounds, vibrations, biological rhythms, and pulse for the first time. Rhythm is further experienced as the fetus descends the birth canal with rhythmic contractions. At birth, the baby makes their first sound in the form of a cry. In the timeframe of 0–6 months, the child's crying can express their "basic needs, to obtain pleasure, and to prevent or reduce pain," and children also engage in making random sounds with objects (Bruscia, 1991). Between 6 and 24 months of age, the child engages in babbling and begins to intentionally manipulate objects to make sounds. From 2–7 years of age, the child begins to verbally express themself, coordinate movement and sound, express emotion, make stories, and keep a rhythm. From ages 7–12, the child may experience formal music lessons and is typically able to employ more fine-tuned sensorimotor movements. Between ages 12 and 18, the child may engage in rebellion against rules and music can provide an outlet for this kind of expression and identity formation. Finally, Bruscia states that from ages 18 and beyond, people can decide "where music fits into their lives."

Dance and Movement Development

Movement starts in the womb and continues throughout life. Some of the earliest noticeable movements in the first few weeks after birth are the newborn reflexes known as muscle reactions, involuntary movements, or neurological reactions to stimulations. These reflexes, including the Moro or Startle Reflex, the Rooting Reflex, the Sucking Reflex, the Tonic Neck Reflex, the Grasp Reflex, the Babinski Reflex, and the Stepping Reflex, are indicators of proper functioning of the baby's nervous system and are crucial for survival. Existing developmental theories in the field of dance/movement therapy build on these earliest movements and are outlined below.

According to Bartenieff (Hackney, 1998), breath underlies all movement and, when integrated throughout the body, will steer at least some body part movements in coordination with the inhale and exhale. Other principles outlined by Bartenieff were movement patterns, increasing in complexity from the most basic ones, such as naval-distal, and mouthing, to more complex ones, including head-tail, upper-lower, homolateral, and contralateral. Bartenieff emphasized that these patterns occurred at every level, from lying to crawling, standing, and walking. She also claimed that the developmental progression was not linear but wavelike. Another movement theorist, Bonnie Bainbridge Cohen (2012), concurred with this sentiment and posed that development overlaps itself with each stage containing elements of all previous stages. She also emphasized that, while reflexes may support movement, they are not actually what drives the movement; instead, an intention affects movement behaviors from the beginning of life. Fundamental locomotor patterns, as per Cohen (2012), underlie all future gross motor coordination, learning, and development, and progress as follows: creeping, crawling, walking, running, jumping, galloping, sliding, hopping, leaping, and lastly skipping, a pattern that requires contralateral integration and occurs around age 6.

The two underlying basic movement patterns of shape-flow, growing, and shrinking, are noticeable from birth and even in utero. In the first year of life and with the horizontal dimension dominating, widening (a growing structure) and narrowing (a shrinking structure) can represent feelings of expanding and comfort or self-containment. A balance between these two structures can promote a feeling of trust (Kestenberg Amighi et al., 2018). In the vertical dimension, during the second year, lengthening (growing structure) serves the feelings of elation and feeling big, while shortening (shrinking structure) structures feeling small and compact. A balance between these two structures can lead to a feeling of stability and the ability to achieve secure standing. In the third year of life, the sagittal dimension (forward/backward) dominates. Here, bulging (growing structure) serves the expression of fullness and completion, and hollowing (shrinking structure) expresses depletion. When a balance is reached between these two structures, the child can develop the feeling of confidence.

The stages of artistic development in art, music, and dance have been found to exist in children around the world even though there might be variations in ages based on the context of development. In addition to these creative aspects of development, an active, unique, and defining component of childhood that is relevant to healthy development is the role of play and imagination. Play is not just leisure, rather it is an essential catalyst of learning and mastery for children.

Stages of Play

Play is a pivotal developmental act for children that allows them to conceptualize the world and how to orient themselves in it (Landreth, 2012). As seen in previous development stages, play too follows of trajectory of focus on the self to increasing awareness of others. Bettelheim, who explored fairytales in relation to child development writes: "just because ... life is often bewildering to (them), the child needs even more to be given the chance to understand (them) self in this complex world with which s/he must learn to copy" (Bettelheim, 1975/1976, p. 5). Explorative play also allows the child to make sense of uncertainties (Russ, 2016). Through play and exploration, children gain insights and solutions that are meaningful to them at their developmental level and the milestones they need to reach (Singha et al., 2020, Russ, 2016). Play provides safety and an opportunity for exploration and joy.

Parten (1932) posed a social theory of play that is still considered a significant theory on children's social participation in play. She observed that the communication between children during play increases as they age. Parten (1932) identified six stages children go through until they reach the age of 5: unoccupied, solitary, spectator, parallel, associative, and cooperative play. The first stage a child goes through is the unoccupied play. The child starts to observe their surroundings and engage in random movements, although they do not yet physically engage with objects. In solitary play, the child plays independently with toys that are not related to the ones other children are playing with. The child is not interested in what others are doing and is absorbed solely by the solitary play activity (Parten, 1932). As Parten (1932) describes, in parallel play, children play beside other children, rather than with each other. They are often attracted to similar toys and naturally gather next to each other, although they do not attempt to manipulate each other's play activity. Although not as socially advanced as cooperative play, parallel play is not as isolated as unoccupied play. Spectator or onlooker play happens when the child deliberately observes the other children play, although they do not yet take active part in the activity. In spectator play, the child chooses groups of people and behavior to observe. Associative play is a group play in which children are interested in other members of the group, even though they are not yet engaged in a cooperative play activity and their behaviors are not in sync with each other. Finally, in cooperative play, children take on roles in the group and engage in a more organized play. Parten's findings were revisited in later publications, and Smith (1978) suggested that some children may skip the parallel play and move directly from solitary play to group play while older children who successfully contribute to group play may also go into short periods of solitary play as a coping behavior. For social play, inclusion of children will vary across contexts, as some children limit their play with others deemed to be different, such as children with disabilities (Diamond, Hong, & Tu, 2008).

Smilansky (1968) identified four phases of play: functional play, constructive play, symbolic/fantasy play, and games with rules. Functional play is identified as basic movements exercised with or in the absence of a play object. Constructive play is a deliberate attempt to create something by using play objects. Dramatic play is when the child uses pretend play to create a situation to fulfill their needs or desires. Finally, games with rules happens when the child understands the pre-set rules in games (Smilansky, 1968).

Play has been a tool employed by therapists since the early 1900s to analyze a child's behavior and access their unconscious by encouraging the expression of fears, desires, and defenses (Klein, 1955). Play does not only help the therapist to understand the inner life of the child, but it also fosters a secure relationship between the child and the therapist (Landreth, 2012). Inspired by the person-centered therapy approach, non-directive Play Therapy was developed by Carl Roger's student, Virginia Axline (1969). In this child-led counseling method, the child is given the chance to express their feelings and difficult thoughts through play in a safe and non-judgmental environment where children's behavior is not controlled or changed (Axline, 1969). Thus, the play therapy experience is an opportunity for the child to freely "play out [their] feelings, just as in certain types of adult therapy, an individual talks out [their] difficulties" (Axline, 1969).

Key Types of Creativity

Like play, creativity is involved in the normative development of children and youth. There are many different types of creativity defined in current literature, including Big C creativity and small c creativity. Big C creativity is associated with transformative events and acts of groundbreaking innovation and novelty (Csikszentmihalyi, 2013; Runco, 2014). Big C creativity refers to genius-level innovation, and examples of this kind of creativity are few and far between in human history (Kaufman & Beghetto, 2009). Small c creativity on the other hand refers to the problem-solving skills of everyday. For example, small c creativity manifests when we put together a creative meal from random ingredients in the kitchen. In the case of children, Vygotsky (1978) suggested that a child pretending to be a mother to a doll, a teacher to their peers, or a driver steering a wheel are all examples of how early play is a manifestation of genuine creativity, as creativity is inherent to pretending. Runco and Jaeger (2012) defined the characteristics of creativity as being novelty and usefulness. Russ (2016) suggests that very often in the case of children their works and approaches might be novel but are not necessarily useful because their creative explorations are part of play and learning. Creating with novelty and usefulness develops over time and with emerging maturity children can create things of meaning and usefulness in the world.

As seen above, children's development is a complex interplay of their own genetic and natural environments that are concurrently shaped and influenced by their interactions in the world. Their natural proclivities in the physical, socio-emotional, cognitive, and artistic domains influence how they develop, their sense of self in relationships, and their sense of their own place in creative pursuits, play, and eventual place in society.

Index